P9-ECZ-623

Most tobacco users are unaware of the harms caused by tobacco use.

Up to half of all tobacco users will die from a tobacco-related disease.

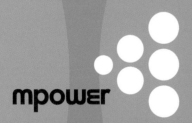

Monitor   Monitor tobacco use and prevention policies

Protect   Protect people from tobacco smoke

Offer   Offer help to quit tobacco use

Warn   Warn about the dangers of tobacco

Enforce   Enforce bans on tobacco advertising, promotion and sponsorship

Raise   Raise taxes on tobacco

Large graphic health warning labels on tobacco packaging and hard-hitting mass media campaigns reduce tobacco use.

WHO Report on the Global Tobacco Epidemic, 2011: Warning about the dangers of tobacco is the third in a series of WHO reports that tracks the status of the tobacco epidemic and the impact of interventions implemented to stop it.

WHO Library Cataloguing-in-Publication Data

WHO report on the global tobacco epidemic, 2011: warning about the dangers of tobacco.

1.Smoking - prevention and control. 2.Tobacco smoke pollution - prevention and control. 3.Tobacco control campaigns. 4.Health policy. I.World Health Organization.

ISBN 978 92 4 156426 7   (NLM classification: WM 290)
ISBN 978 92 4 068781 3 (pdf)
ISBN 978 92 4 068782 0 (epub)
ISBN 978 92 4 068783 7 (mobi)

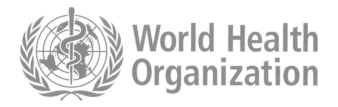

World Health Organization

WHO REPORT ON THE GLOBAL TOBACCO EPIDEMIC, 2011

Warning about the dangers of tobacco

Made possible by funding from Bloomberg Philanthropies

Contents

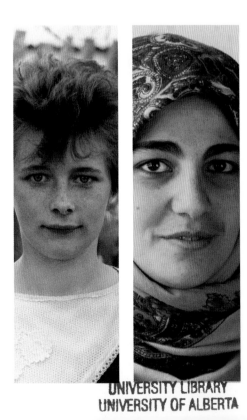
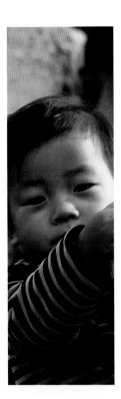
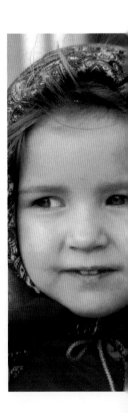

Appendices IV through X are available in electronic format on the CD accompanying this book and online at http://www.who.int/tobacco/

ABBREVIATIONS

AFR	WHO African Region
AMR	WHO Region of the Americas
CDC	Centers for Disease Control and Prevention
COP	Conference of the Parties to the WHO FCTC
EMR	WHO Eastern Mediterranean Region
EUR	WHO European Region
NRT	nicotine replacement therapy
SEAR	WHO South-East Asia Region
STEPS	WHO's STEPwise approach to Surveillance
US$	United States dollar
WHO	World Health Organization
WHO FCTC	WHO Framework Convention on Tobacco Control
WHO TFI	WHO Tobacco Free Initiative
WPR	WHO Western Pacific Region

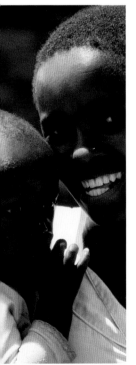
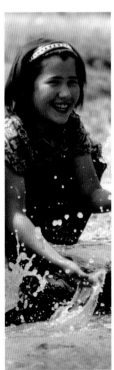
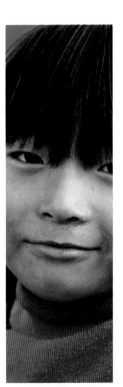
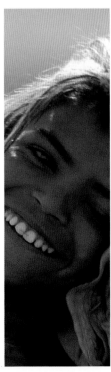

Over the past two years, 1.1 billion people have become covered by at least one MPOWER measure newly applied at the highest level.

People have an inherent right to receive information about the health dangers of tobacco use, and countries have an obligation to provide it.

Dr Ala Alwan, Assistant Director-General, World Health Organization

PROGRESS CONTINUES – NEARLY 3.8 BILLION PEOPLE ARE NOW COVERED BY AN EFFECTIVE TOBACCO CONTROL MEASURE

The number of people now protected by tobacco control measures is growing at a remarkable pace. The progress made on applying measures that reduce the demand for tobacco is a sign of the increasing impact of the WHO Framework Convention on Tobacco Control, which continues to be one of the most rapidly embraced, measurably successful treaties in United Nations history.

This report, the third periodic country-level examination of the global tobacco epidemic, identifies the countries that have applied effective tobacco control measures that save lives. These countries can be held up as models of action for the many countries that need to do more to protect their people from the harms of tobacco use. Tobacco continues to kill nearly 6 million people each year, including more than 600 000 non-smokers who die from exposure to tobacco smoke. Up to half of the world's 1 billion smokers will eventually die of a tobacco-related disease. However, we have the power to change these circumstances.

Over the past two years, 1.1 billion people have become covered by at least one MPOWER measure newly applied at the highest level. This is the result of action taken by 30 countries – over half of them classified as low- or middle-income – which have applied measures that, while requiring relatively little investment, are proven to be highly effective at changing tobacco use patterns and saving lives.

The focus of this report is on warning people about the harms of tobacco use. People have an inherent right to receive this information, and countries have an obligation to provide it. The two main types of warnings are examined: health warning labels on tobacco packages and national anti-tobacco mass media campaigns. Large and graphic warning labels and hard-hitting mass media campaigns have proven effective in reducing tobacco use and encouraging people to quit. This report presents for the first time

detailed national-level data collected on a global basis for anti-tobacco mass media campaigns.

The data are impressive. More than 1 billion people now live in countries with legislation that requires large graphic health warnings on every cigarette pack sold in their countries, and 1.9 billion people live in the 23 countries that have aired high-quality national anti-tobacco mass media campaigns within the past two years. It is clear that substantial progress is being made against this deadly product. Low- and middle-income countries have been in the forefront of developing anti-tobacco mass media campaigns, showing that countries can successfully implement this intervention regardless of income classification.

Nevertheless, the tobacco epidemic continues to expand because of ongoing tobacco industry marketing, population growth in countries where tobacco use is increasing, and the extreme addictiveness of tobacco that makes it difficult for people to stop smoking once they start. Although there has been progress, only 19 countries follow best-practice standards by requiring large graphic health warnings on tobacco product packages – none of which are low-income countries. All countries, in partnership with the United Nations, health development agencies and civil society, can and must do more by meeting their commitments under the WHO Framework Convention on Tobacco Control and its corresponding guidelines.

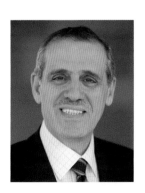

This report appears at a crucial moment in the fight against the growing epidemic of noncommunicable diseases (NCDs) – primarily cancers, diabetes, and cardiovascular and chronic lung diseases – which account for 63% of all deaths worldwide and for which tobacco use is one of the biggest contributing agents. These diseases kill an astounding 36 million people each year, with 80% of deaths occurring in low- and middle-income countries that can least afford them. An estimated 9 million deaths occur below the age of 60 years. On 19–20 September 2011, the United Nations General Assembly will hold its first-ever high-level meeting to consider the threat and impact of noncommunicable diseases on global health and human development. Heads of State will discuss during this meeting in New York how to raise awareness of and plot strategies against this cluster of related diseases that share several risk factors, most notably tobacco use.

Because tobacco use and exposure to tobacco smoke cause a large proportion of global illness and death, tobacco control must be given the high priority it deserves so that we can expand on the successes we have already realized. Consequently, tobacco control measures are expected to be scaled up as a core component of the outcome for the United Nations high-level meeting on NCD's.

As Dr Margaret Chan, Director-General of the World Health Organization has said, "What gets measured gets done". This report is a strong and important step in our ongoing measurement of what has been achieved in tobacco control and how much more countries need to do. We can and must continue this work – millions of people's lives are at stake.

Dr Ala Alwan
Assistant Director-General
World Health Organization

Summary

Tobacco use continues to be the leading global cause of preventable death. It kills nearly 6 million people and causes hundreds of billions of dollars of economic damage worldwide each year. Most of these deaths occur in low- and middle-income countries, and this disparity is expected to widen further over the next several decades. If current trends continue, by 2030 tobacco will kill more than 8 million people worldwide each year, with 80% of these premature deaths among people living in low- and middle-income countries. Over the course of the 21st century, tobacco use could kill a billion people or more unless urgent action is taken.

The World Health Organization Framework Convention on Tobacco Control (WHO FCTC) demonstrates global political will to strengthen tobacco control and save lives. The WHO FCTC is a legally binding global treaty that provides the foundation for countries to implement and manage tobacco control programmes to address the growing epidemic of tobacco use. As of May 2011, the WHO FCTC has 173 Parties covering 87% of the world's population, making it one of the most rapidly embraced treaties in United Nations history.

To help countries fulfil their WHO FCTC obligations, in 2008 WHO introduced the MPOWER package of six evidence-based tobacco control measures that are proven to reduce tobacco use and save lives. The MPOWER measures provide practical assistance with country-level implementation of effective policies to reduce the demand for tobacco. The MPOWER measures focus on demand reduction, although WHO also recognizes the importance of and is committed to implementing the supply-side measures contained in the WHO FCTC.

The continued success of the WHO FCTC is detailed in this year's *WHO Report on the Global Tobacco Epidemic, 2011*, the third in the series of WHO reports on the status of global tobacco control policy achievement. All data on the level of countries' achievement for the six MPOWER measures have been updated through 2010, and additional data have been collected on warning the public about the dangers of tobacco. This year's report examines in detail the two primary strategies to provide health warnings – labels on tobacco product packaging and anti-tobacco mass media campaigns. The report provides a comprehensive overview of the evidence base for warning people about the harms of tobacco use, as well as country-specific information on the status of these measures.

To continue the process of improving data analysis, categories of policy achievement

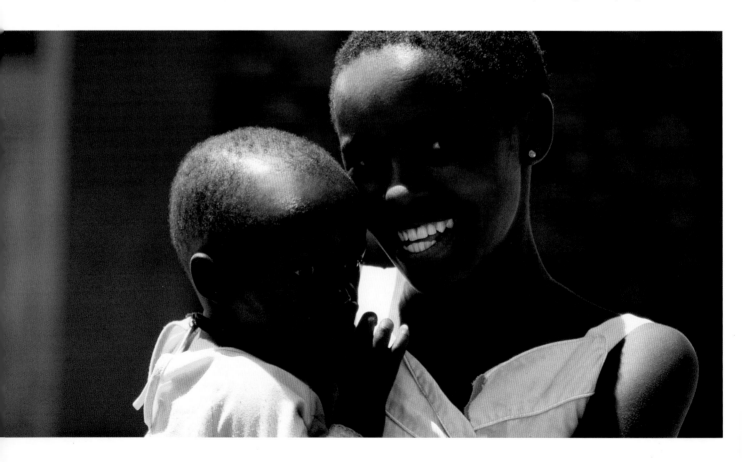

19 countries with more than a billion people now have pack warning laws at the highest level of achievement in this policy area.

have been refined and, where possible, made consistent with new and evolving WHO FCTC guidelines. Data from the 2009 report have been reanalysed to be consistent with these new categories, allowing for more direct comparisons of the data across both reports. This year continues the practice of printing a streamlined summary version of the report and publishing more detailed country-specific data online (http://www.who.int/tobacco).

Substantial progress continues to be made in applying the MPOWER measures. Roughly 3.8 billion people (55% of the world's population) are covered by at least one measure at the highest level of achievement, including 1.1 billion people covered by a new policy since 2008. More than 1 billion people (17% of the world's population)

are covered by two or more measures at the highest level of achievement. Gains were made in all areas, with a total of 30 countries enacting at least one new MPOWER measure at the highest level since 2008. Anti-tobacco mass media campaigns, an MPOWER measure assessed for the first time for this report, occurred in 23 countries reaching 1.9 billion people during 2009 and 2010.

Together, health warning labels and anti-tobacco mass media campaigns are the most widely embraced MPOWER measures, based on population coverage. The MPOWER measure showing the largest progress since the 2009 report, based on population coverage, is provision of health warning labels on tobacco packaging. More than

a billion people now have pack warning laws at the highest level of achievement in this policy area, a gain of three countries (with nearly half a billion people) that have passed such legislation within the past two years. Notably, the United States of America will move from very weak warning label requirements to among the world's strongest in 2012, when its new warning label regulations are scheduled to be implemented.

This year's report also provides, for the first time ever, systematically collected information about anti-tobacco mass media campaigns, a highly effective method of warning the public about the dangers of tobacco. The data reveal the promising work being done in this area – more than

SHARE OF THE WORLD POPULATION COVERED BY SELECTED TOBACCO CONTROL POLICIES, 2010

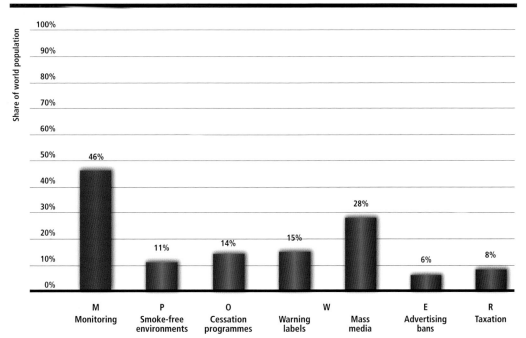

Note: The tobacco control policies depicted here correspond to the highest level of achievement at the national level; for the definitions of these highest categories refer to Technical Note I.

1.9 billion people (28% of the world's population) live in the 23 countries that ran at least one strong anti-tobacco mass media campaign during the reporting period. Only seven of the 23 countries that ran a strong campaign are classified as high-income – the majority reporting exemplary campaigns are low- or middle-income countries, providing evidence that all countries, regardless of income level, can run effective mass media campaigns.

The *WHO Report on the Global Tobacco Epidemic, 2009* focused on the importance of protecting the public from the dangers of second-hand tobacco smoke through comprehensive smoke-free laws. Substantial gains have been made in this area since 2008 – 16 additional countries have passed national legislation that bans smoking in all public places and workplaces, including bars and restaurants, with the result that over 385 million people have been newly protected from the health harms of tobacco smoke. An additional 100 million people are protected by comprehensive smoke-free laws that have been passed at the subnational level since 2008.

As countries continue to build on the progress achieved since becoming Parties to the WHO FCTC, more people are being protected from the harms of second-hand tobacco smoke, provided with help to quit tobacco use, exposed to effective health warnings through tobacco package labelling and mass media campaigns, protected against tobacco industry marketing tactics and covered by taxation policies designed to decrease tobacco use and fund tobacco control and other health programmes. Perseverance by all countries in expanding the reach of tobacco control programmes is needed to achieve the goal of a tobacco-free world, and is critical to saving the lives of the billion people who may otherwise die from tobacco-related illness this century.

More than 1.9 billion people live in the 23 countries that ran at least one strong anti-tobacco mass media campaign during the reporting period.

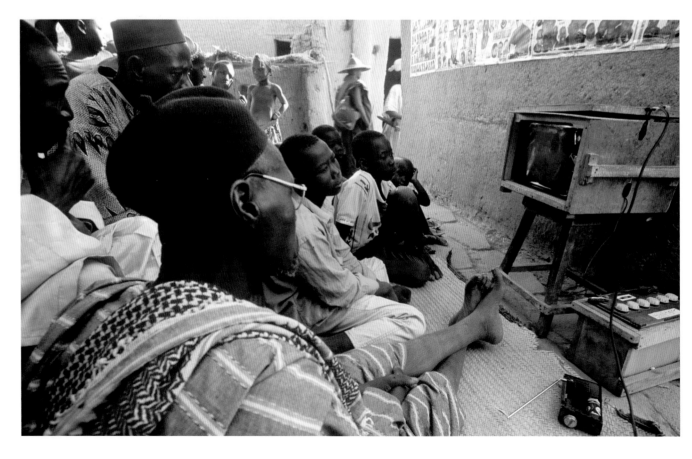

THE STATE OF SELECTED TOBACCO CONTROL POLICIES IN THE WORLD, 2010

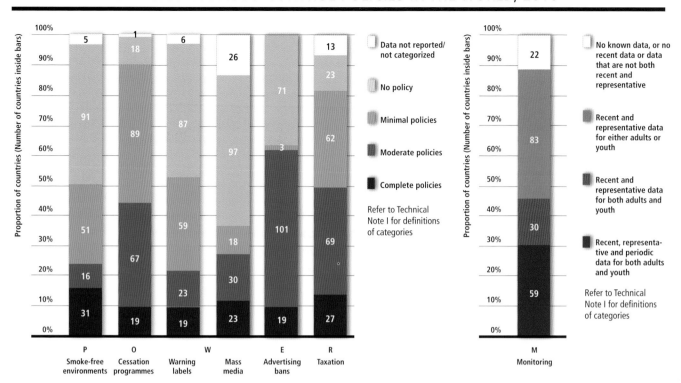

Proportion of countries (Number of countries inside bars)
100%
90%
80%
70%
60%
50%
40%
30%
20%
10%
0%
5
91
51
16
31
1
18
89
67
19
6
87
59
23
19
26
97
18
30
23
71
3
101
19
13
23
62
69
27
P
Smoke-free environments
O
Cessation programmes
W
Warning labels
Mass media
E
Advertising bans
R
Taxation
Data not reported/ not categorized
No policy
Minimal policies
Moderate policies
Complete policies
Refer to Technical Note I for definitions of categories
22
83
30
59
M
Monitoring
No known data, or no recent data or data that are not both recent and representative
Recent and representative data for either adults or youth
Recent and representative data for both adults and youth
Recent, representative and periodic data for both adults and youth
Refer to Technical Note I for definitions of categories

INCREASE IN THE SHARE OF THE WORLD POPULATION COVERED BY SELECTED TOBACCO CONTROL POLICIES SINCE 2008

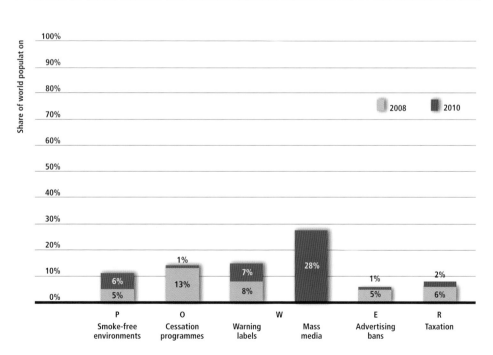

Share of world populat on
100%
90%
80%
70%
60%
50%
40%
30%
20%
10%
0%
2008
2010
6%
5%
1%
13%
7%
8%
28%
1%
5%
2%
6%
P
Smoke-free environments
O
Cessation programmes
W
Warning labels
Mass media
E
Advertising bans
R
Taxation

Notes: Changes of less than 1% are not labelled on the graph.
Data on monitoring are not shown in this graph because they are not comparable between 2008 and 2010. Mass media data were collected for the first time in 2010, so no comparable data are shown for 2008. The tobacco control policies depicted here correspond to the highest level of achievement at the national level; for the definitions of these highest categories refer to Technical Note I.

WHO Framework Convention on Tobacco Control

When WHO was established in 1948, its Member States incorporated the power to negotiate treaties into its Constitution. This power remained dormant until 1996, when the World Health Assembly adopted a resolution requesting the WHO Director-General to initiate development of a framework convention for global tobacco control in accordance with the WHO Constitution. This unprecedented request was made in response to the rapid globalization of the tobacco epidemic and the growing magnitude of the health burden associated with tobacco use, which kills nearly 6 million people and causes hundreds of billions of dollars in economic damage worldwide every year.

Today, the WHO Framework Convention on Tobacco Control (WHO FCTC) (1) is one of the most rapidly embraced treaties in the history of the United Nations, with 173 Parties covering 87% of the world's population. It contains legally binding obligations for its Parties, addresses the need to reduce both demand for and supply of tobacco, and provides a comprehensive direction for implementing tobacco control policy at all levels of government. The treaty's governing body is the Conference of the Parties (COP), an intergovernmental entity composed of all Parties with responsibility for guiding and promoting effective implementation of the WHO FCTC. As part of this responsibility, the COP considers the reports submitted periodically by each Party, in accordance with Article 21 of the treaty, and the global summary prepared by the Convention Secretariat to review the progress, successes and challenges of implementation.

To reflect the complexities of the tobacco epidemic, as well as the challenge of countering a very well-funded and powerful multinational industry, WHO FCTC negotiators included broad, encompassing treaty provisions to address demand reduction and supply reduction issues in Articles 6 and 8–17:

Article 6. Price and tax measures to reduce the demand for tobacco.
Article 8. Protection from exposure to tobacco smoke.
Article 9. Regulation of the contents of tobacco products.
Article 10. Regulation of tobacco product disclosures.
Article 11. Packaging and labelling of tobacco products.
Article 12. Education, communication, training and public awareness.

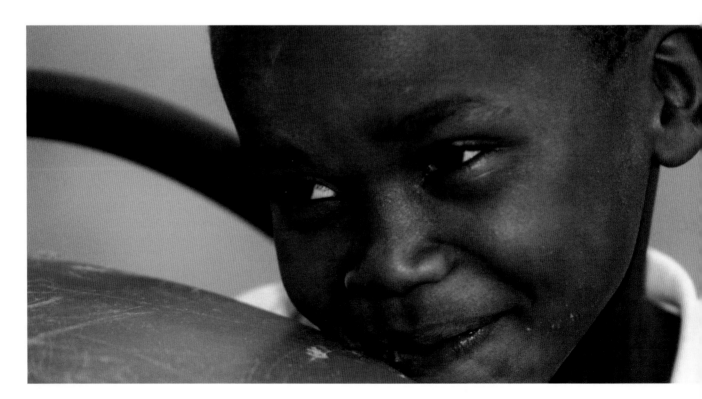

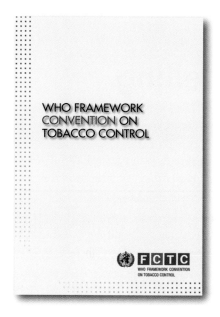

WHO FRAMEWORK CONVENTION ON TOBACCO CONTROL

Article 13. Tobacco advertising, promotion and sponsorship.
Article 14. Reduction measures concerning tobacco dependence and cessation.
Article 15. Illicit trade in tobacco products.
Article 16. Sales to and by minors.
Article 17. Provision of support for economically viable alternative activities.

In addition to these supply and demand measures, the WHO FCTC provides guidance and encouragement for collaboration in implementation; in particular, sections addressing General obligations (Article 5), Scientific and technical cooperation and communication of information (Articles 20, 21 and 22) and International cooperation and resources (Articles 25 and 26) help Parties maximize best practices, share experiences and avoid interference from the tobacco industry.

The text of the WHO FCTC, and the success in implementing effective national and global tobacco control policies since its entry into force, demonstrates strong international commitment to ending the tobacco epidemic. The treaty establishes standards that underpin and drive tobacco control throughout the world and reinforces the role and strength of international law as a tool to prevent disease and disability. The power of this treaty lies not only in its obligations, which are binding for all Parties, but also in the formal demonstration of the need, recognized globally, to "protect present and future generations from the devastating health, social, environmental and economic consequences of tobacco consumption and exposure to tobacco smoke" (1).

In Article 7 (Non-price measures to reduce the demand for tobacco), the WHO FCTC mandates: "Each Party shall adopt and implement effective legislative, executive, administrative or other measures necessary to implement its obligations pursuant to Articles 8 to 13 … The Conference of the Parties shall propose appropriate guidelines for the implementation of the provisions of these Articles" (1).

The COP unanimously adopted guidelines for Article 11 in November 2008 and unanimously adopted Article 12 guidelines in November 2010. These guidelines establish high standards of accountability for treaty compliance and include clear statements of purpose, objectives and guiding principles.

Many countries can easily improve policies by increasing the size of warning labels, strengthening the wording of warnings and making them more specific, and including pictures rather than text-only warnings.

Article 11 – Packaging and labelling of tobacco products

The WHO FCTC is an evidence-based treaty: nowhere is this more clear than in Article 11, which sets out strong, clear and legally obligatory standards for health warning labels on tobacco packaging. These standards are derived from strong data that health warnings encourage tobacco users to quit and help keep young people from starting. Article 11 forms the basis for international action to communicate the health risks of tobacco, and requires all Parties to implement compliant warning labels on all tobacco products sold or otherwise distributed within their jurisdictions within three years after entry into force of the treaty for that Party.

Article 11 of the WHO FCTC requires that health warning labels on tobacco packaging (2):

- be approved by the competent national authority;
- should cover 50% or more of the principal pack display areas, but should be no less than 30%;
- be large, clear, visible and legible;
- not use misleading terms like "light" and "mild";
- be rotated periodically to remain fresh and novel to consumers;
- display information on relevant constituents and emissions of tobacco products as defined by national authorities;
- appear in the principal language(s) of the country.

The strength of the language and of the obligations set forth in Article 11 have led to measurable global progress in providing people with effective warnings about the dangers of tobacco, although there is still work to be done in most countries and in all regions. Many countries can easily improve policies by increasing the size of warning labels, strengthening the wording of warnings and making them more specific, and including pictures rather than text-only warnings.

WHO FCTC health warnings database

In order to promote international cooperation, the COP requested that WHO's Tobacco Free Initiative (TFI) establish and maintain a central database of pictorial health warnings and messages. TFI, in collaboration with the WHO FCTC Convention Secretariat, has established such a database to facilitate sharing of pictorial health warnings and messages among countries and Parties.* This type of assistance and support are part of WHO's larger tobacco control programme driven by the WHO FCTC. To provide technical assistance to help Member States fulfil some of their commitments to the treaty, WHO has proposed the MPOWER package of measures. MPOWER supports the implementation of six effective tobacco control measures proven to reduce tobacco use. Each measure reflects one or more provisions of the WHO FCTC, and the package of six measures is an important entry point for scaling up efforts to reduce the demand for tobacco. MPOWER is an integral part of the WHO Action Plan for the Prevention and Control of Noncommunicable Diseases (3), which was endorsed at the 61st World Health Assembly in 2008 and reflects the commitment of WHO Member States to the implementation of the WHO FCTC.

* The health warnings database is freely accessible to the public at: http://www.who.int/tobacco/healthwarningsdatabase/en/index.html

Guidelines for implementation of Article 11

The purpose of the Article 11 guidelines is to assist Parties in meeting their WHO FCTC obligations and to suggest means by which Parties can increase the effectiveness of their packaging and labelling measures. The substance of the Article 11 guidelines is separated into seven sections (2).

Developing effective packaging and labelling requirements

The Article 11 guidelines articulate recommendations on design elements of effective warning labels and display of information on constituents and emissions, and encourage the following measures to increase the effectiveness of packaging and labelling (2).

- Warning labels should cover as much of the principal display areas as possible.
- If used, pictures should be in full colour.
- Warnings should appear on the front and back of packs, as well as at the top of principal display areas, to maximize their visibility and in such a way that the opening of the package does not permanently damage or conceal the warning.
- Parties should consider printing warnings on cigarette filters and/or on other related materials (e.g. packages of cigarette tubes, filters and papers) as well as other instruments (e.g. those used for water pipe smoking).
- Warnings should address different issues related to tobacco use, in addition to harmful health effects and the impact of second-hand tobacco smoke exposure (e.g. Advice on cessation, the addictive nature of tobacco, adverse economic and social outcomes such as the annual cost of purchasing tobacco products, the impact of tobacco use on others, adverse environmental outcomes, and tobacco industry practices).
- Warnings may be designed to target subgroups (e.g. youth).
- Warnings should not contain quantitative or qualitative statements about tobacco constituents and emissions (e.g. tar, nicotine and carbon monoxide figures) that might imply that one brand is less harmful than another.
- Where possible, warnings should undergo pre-market testing to assess their effectiveness with the intended target population.
- Parties should look to pack warnings used elsewhere for best-practice examples on how to implement this intervention.
- Where quit line services are available, quit line numbers can be included on warning labels to improve linkage to cessation services.
- Parties should consider legislation to mandate plain, generic packaging and prohibit or restrict the use of logos, colours, brand images or promotional information.

Process for developing effective packaging and labelling requirements

Warning labels should appear on all tobacco packaging, and those labels should be effective in accurately conveying the health risks of smoking. This section of the guidelines addresses considerations that each Party must take into account to accomplish this.

Developing effective packaging and labelling restrictions

Tobacco packaging should not be misleading. The guidelines specifically recommend that figures for emission yields not be included on tobacco packages, and that Parties consider plain, generic packaging that restricts the use of logos, brand images and promotional information by limiting packaging only to brand names and product names displayed in a standard colour and font style.

Legal measures

To assist Parties in generating and implementing enforceable measures that satisfy WHO FCTC requirements, the guidelines include a number of specific recommendations on drafting legislation to ensure that effective warning labels are included on all tobacco products.

Enforcement

Appropriate infrastructure and budget are critical to enforcement. Parties should ensure that all stakeholders are aware of new labelling measures and use inspectors or agents to conduct spot checks at import, export and retail facilities. Reactions to noncompliance must be rapid and, if possible, the public should be empowered to report noncompliance and file complaints.

Monitoring and evaluating packaging and labelling measures

Monitoring and evaluating the effects of tobacco control measures are critical to assess their impact, identify where improvements are needed, and add to the body of best-practice evidence. The guidelines note that monitoring and evaluation are ongoing processes.

International cooperation

The guidelines note that international cooperation is needed to maximize the effectiveness of packing and labelling provisions. The WHO FCTC provides for and promotes cooperation, information and expertise exchange, and support between and among Parties in several areas.

Article 12 – Education, communication, training and public awareness

Understanding that even the most effective warning labels are not sufficient, Article 12 of the WHO FCTC contains obligations for Parties to promote and strengthen public awareness of tobacco control issues through other means. Article 12 requires Parties to provide the public with widely accessible and comprehensive information on the addictiveness of tobacco and the risks and harms of tobacco consumption and exposure to tobacco smoke, as well as the adverse health, economic and environmental consequences of tobacco production. Parties are also required to give the public access to a wide range of information on the tobacco industry.

Education, communication and training are most effective when incorporated into a comprehensive tobacco control programme.

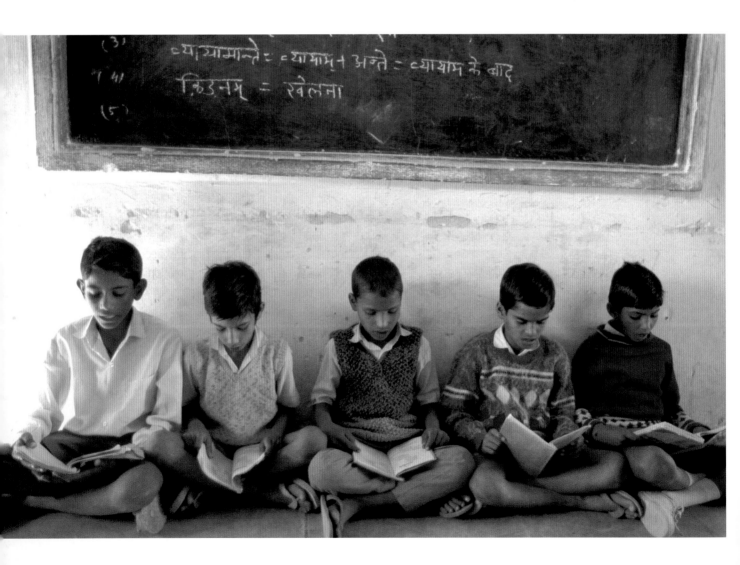

Guidelines for implementation of Article 12

The objectives of the Article 12 guidelines are to identify key measures needed to successfully educate, communicate with and train people on the health, social, economic and environmental consequences of tobacco production and consumption and of exposure to tobacco smoke, and to guide Parties in establishing a sustainable infrastructure needed to support these measures. As with other WHO FCTC guidelines, these draw on the best available evidence, best practices and experience. The guidelines also articulate a set of guiding principles for implementation. The substance of the Article 12 guidelines falls into six sections (4):

Providing an infrastructure to raise public awareness

The guidelines emphasize that effectively raising public awareness requires solid, sustainable infrastructure that should include a tobacco control focal point within the national government to catalyse, coordinate and facilitate delivery of tobacco-related education, communication and training programmes, and to monitor and evaluate these programmes.

Running effective education, communication and training programmes

The guidelines provide definitions of key terms relevant to awareness raising as well as tactics for Parties to implement effective strategies. These definitions emphasize that education, communication and training are most effective when incorporated into a comprehensive tobacco control programme, and that they require a sustainable approach to maintain effectiveness.

Involving civil society

Parties are encouraged to actively involve civil society in planning, developing, implementing, monitoring and evaluating tobacco control education, communication and training programmes. Governments should also identify and involve key community tobacco control leadership and consider providing direct financial or other support to tobacco control efforts undertaken by civil society.

Ensuring wide access to information on the tobacco industry

The guidelines outline the many strategies employed by the tobacco industry to undermine tobacco control, and reference the obligation under WHO FCTC Article 5.3 to ensure that policies are free from tobacco industry influence. To be effective, tobacco control education, communication and training require accurate and truthful information about the tobacco industry; in turn, Parties are required to make such information freely and readily accessible to the public.

Strengthening international cooperation

The guidelines recognize the importance of sharing information and best practices between and among countries as well as the importance of collaborating to raise global public awareness of tobacco control.

Monitoring of implementation and revision of the guidelines

The guidelines emphasize the need for Parties to monitor, evaluate and revise their communication, education and training measures to facilitate comparisons, observe trends and provide clear goals for implementation. Evaluation should also include determination of need, formulation of objectives and identification of resources required before initiating awareness raising programmes.

Additionally, 10 annexes are appended to the Article 12 guidelines that provide practical ideas for implementation. These annexes are a series of lists, including checklists for an action plan for implementation of education, communication and training activities within a comprehensive tobacco control programme, and for research-based strategies and programmes. Eight additional lists follow these checklists and cover specific public awareness, education and training topic areas.

Warn about the dangers of tobacco

People have a right to accurate information about the harms of tobacco use

Consumers of tobacco products have a fundamental right to accurate information about the risks of smoking and other forms of tobacco use (5). The WHO FCTC recognizes that a basic requisite for reducing tobacco use is that every person be informed of the health consequences, addictive nature, and potential for disability and premature death posed by tobacco consumption and exposure to tobacco smoke.

Education about the dangers of tobacco use and second-hand smoke exposure can influence an individual's decision to start or continue using tobacco. Ultimately, one of the objectives of warning the public about the dangers of tobacco is to change social norms about tobacco use. This will cause many individuals to choose not to use tobacco, and also increase support for other tobacco control measures.

Many people are unaware of the harms of tobacco use

Despite clear evidence about the dangers of tobacco use, many tobacco users worldwide underestimate the full extent of the risk to themselves and others (6). Although a large number of people know in general terms that tobacco use is harmful to their health, many aspects of tobacco use have not been

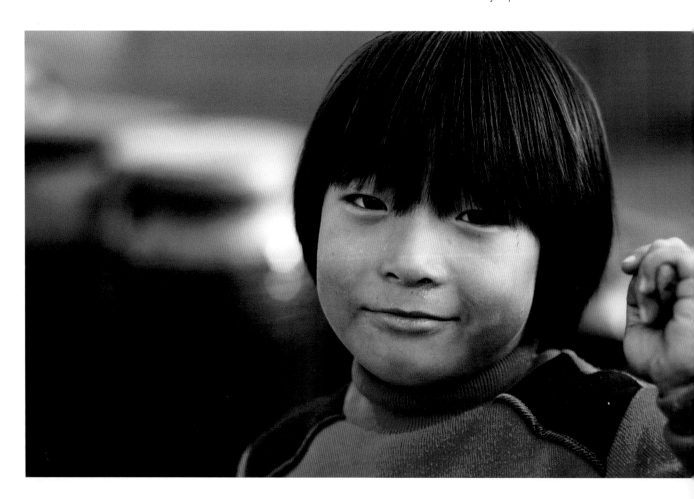

Proven policies to reduce tobacco use include mandatory health warning labels on tobacco packaging and hard-hitting mass media campaigns that show the harms of tobacco use.

adequately explained and as a result are not well understood by most tobacco users.

Many tobacco users are unaware of the harmful chemicals in tobacco products and tobacco smoke, as well as the wide spectrum of specific illnesses caused by tobacco use (7), and frequently do not know that smoking also causes cancers other than lung cancer as well as heart disease, stroke,

and many other diseases (8). Many smokers also incorrectly believe that "light" or "low-tar" cigarettes are less harmful (9–11).

This lack of knowledge leads to a substantial misperception of the risks involved with tobacco use. As a result, smokers tend to grossly underestimate the health risks of tobacco use to themselves and of second-hand smoke exposure to others. Smokers

often do not accurately assess the likelihood of disability and death from long-term tobacco use, or the full extent of harm caused by second-hand smoke exposure. Many non-smokers are also not aware of the dangers of second-hand smoke (12).

The extreme addictive nature of tobacco is also not widely acknowledged. Many people, including smokers, incorrectly

KNOWLEDGE ABOUT THE HARMS OF TOBACCO IS HIGHER IN COUNTRIES WITH TOBACCO PACKAGE WARNINGS

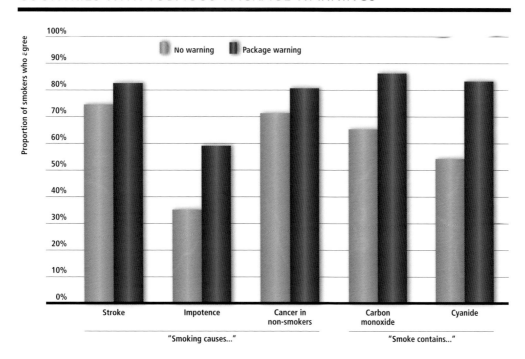

Source: (6).

believe that tobacco use is simply a "bad habit", not an addiction (13). They often do not fully comprehend the speed with which people can become addicted to nicotine, or the degree of addiction, and grossly overestimate the likelihood that they will be able to quit easily when desired and before health problems occur.

Showing the truth about the dangers of tobacco use requires evidence-based health warnings. These warnings should appear directly on tobacco product packaging, be included within tobacco advertising and on marketing materials (where not yet banned), and be contained in anti-tobacco advertisements in various types of media. Proven measures to reduce tobacco use include mandatory health warning labels on

tobacco packaging and hard-hitting mass media campaigns that show the harms of tobacco use (14).

Both youth and adults benefit from adult-focused approaches

Because people are most likely to begin to use tobacco as adolescents (15), it is especially important to inform young people about the harms of tobacco use before they start. Health warnings can be conveyed using many different methods, including warning labels on tobacco packaging and anti-tobacco mass media campaigns. Although there is a prevalent belief that effectively providing youth with warnings

requires approaches different from those used for adults, broad educational efforts that reach all age groups have been shown to be more effective in influencing youth behaviour than efforts targeted specifically at them (16). Anti-tobacco programmes directed at children to keep them from starting tobacco use are politically popular and have broad public appeal, but do not contribute substantially to reducing youth smoking experimentation or initiation when conducted as part of health education classes in schools (17, 18). Focusing anti-tobacco educational initiatives on children could also weaken a more comprehensive population-wide approach that would have a greater long-term impact (19).

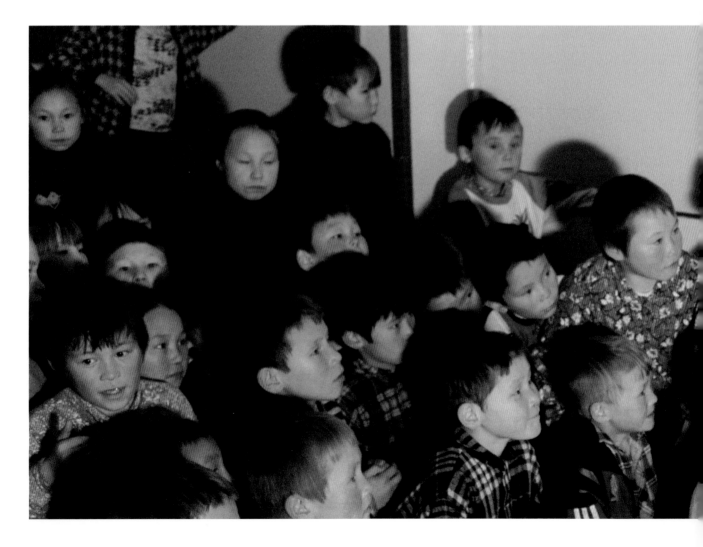

People have a fundamental right to information about the harms of tobacco; countries have a legal obligation to provide it.

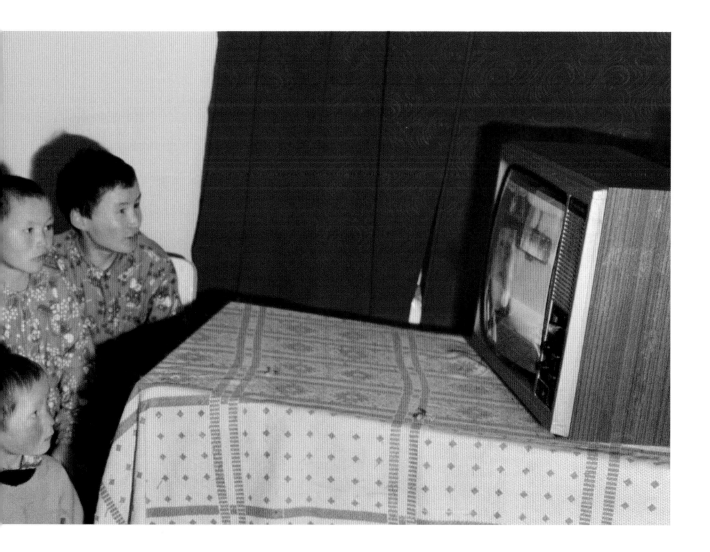

Health warning labels on tobacco packaging

Health warning labels are effective

Effective warning labels on tobacco packaging serve several purposes, including disrupting the marketing value of the packages. Because traditional avenues for marketing tobacco products have become increasingly restricted due to wider adoption of bans on tobacco advertising, promotion and sponsorship, the tobacco industry has become increasingly more reliant on cigarette packaging as a primary marketing vehicle (16, 20, 21). Warning labels reduce the marketing effect of tobacco product packaging, making it more difficult for tobacco companies to reinforce brand awareness.

The maximum reduction in the marketing effect of tobacco packaging would be achieved through the use of generic (i.e. "plain" or "standardized") packaging, which uses only standard type fonts in a single colour on a plain background to provide the minimum information necessary to identify a product, without the use of logos, stylized fonts, colours, designs or images, or any additional descriptive language. Because generic packaging may increase accurate perceptions of the risk of tobacco use and decrease smoking rates (21), efforts to prohibit the use of logos, colours, brand images and other promotional information are gaining traction. The plainer the package and the fewer branding elements included, the less

favourably smokers will perceive the packs and the greater the impact pictorial health warnings may have (22). The Australian Parliament is debating the adoption of a bill to require generic tobacco packaging in 2011, which would make Australia the first country to mandate generic packaging beginning in July 2012.

Warning labels also shift the value of packaging away from marketing and towards public health messaging. Effective warning labels increase smokers' awareness of health risks (6) and increase the likelihood that they will think about cessation and reduce tobacco consumption (23–25). Prominent health warning labels that fully comply with WHO FCTC

Effective warning labels increase smokers' awareness of health risks, and increase the likelihood that smokers will think about cessation and reduce tobacco consumption.

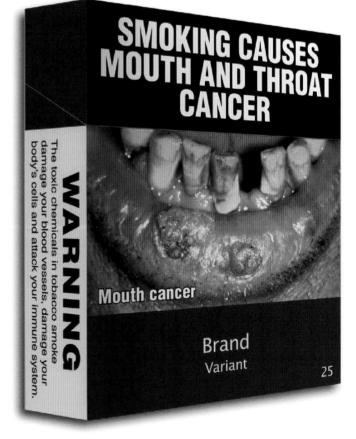

Australian government's proposed design for plain packaging of tobacco products

requirements provide the most direct health messages to smokers (6, 26, 27) and potentially reach smokers every time they purchase or consume tobacco products (28, 29). Warnings are also seen by non-smokers, affecting their perceptions of smoking and decisions about initiation, and ultimately helping to change the image of tobacco and "denormalize" its use (30) (the previous chapter gives details of specific guidelines contained in the WHO FCTC for characteristics of effective warning labels).

Although most of the evidence currently available has examined the impact of health warning labels on the packaging of manufactured cigarettes, pictorial health

warning labels are also effective in reducing the appeal and increasing the perception of risk of smokeless tobacco products among youth (31).

Pictorial warning labels are especially powerful

Pictorial labels are more effective than text-only warnings (6, 28, 32–38), in part because they are noticed by more people, provide more information, and evoke emotional responses to the images (28, 39). Pictorial warnings are even more important in countries with low literacy rates where many people cannot understand written messages. Stronger health warnings tend

to sustain their effects longer than weaker or more general warnings (28). Because smokers recall more readily the warnings they have seen recently (40), it is important to rotate warning labels periodically and to introduce new ones regularly.

Warning labels that include pictures are most likely to be noticed and rated effective by smokers (27, 32), and increasing the size of warning labels also increases their effectiveness (28). The three countries that currently have the largest pictorial health warning requirements for cigarette packages (as an average of the package front and back) are Uruguay (80%), Mauritius (65%) and Mexico (65%).

INTRODUCTION OF GRAPHIC WARNING LABELS IN CANADA INCREASES SMOKERS' INTENTION TO QUIT

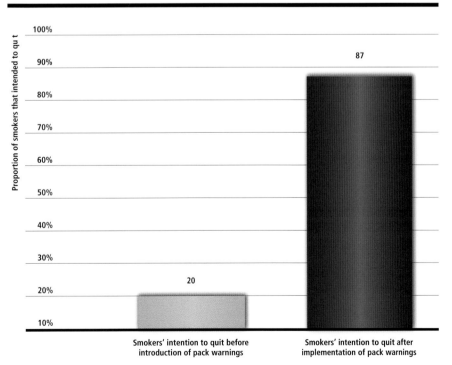

Source: (29).

The size of the warning on the front of the package is most critical for immediate impact, as packs are generally displayed with the front showing and smokers are most likely to take cigarettes from packs while looking at the package front (28). The placement of warning labels at the top of the pack, rather than at the bottom, is also likely to increase their visibility and make it more difficult to conceal the warnings in retail displays.

After Canada became the first country to introduce large, graphic health warning labels on cigarette packages in 2001, smokers who had read, thought about and discussed the labels were more likely to have quit, made a quit attempt, or reduced their smoking (29). About three in 10 former smokers reported that the labels had motivated them to quit and more than a quarter said that labels helped them remain abstinent (41). In another Canadian study, about a fifth of smokers reported reducing their consumption as a result of seeing the pack warning labels (42).

Australia introduced graphic health warning labels in 2006 that caused more than half of smokers to believe that they had an increased risk of dying from smoking-related illness, with 38% feeling motivated to quit (40). Other countries with pictorial warning labels, including Brazil (26), Singapore (43) and Thailand (44), report similar effects on smoking-related behaviour. Graphic warnings also persuade smokers to protect the health of non-smokers by smoking less inside their homes and avoiding smoking near children (43, 45).

Health warning labels can be used to promote quit lines

Smokers are more likely to reduce tobacco consumption and think about quitting as a result of seeing strong graphic warning labels (25). Providing direct information about cessation services on tobacco packaging, in addition to health warnings, may further motivate smokers to make a quit attempt. Promoting quit lines by including telephone numbers directly on

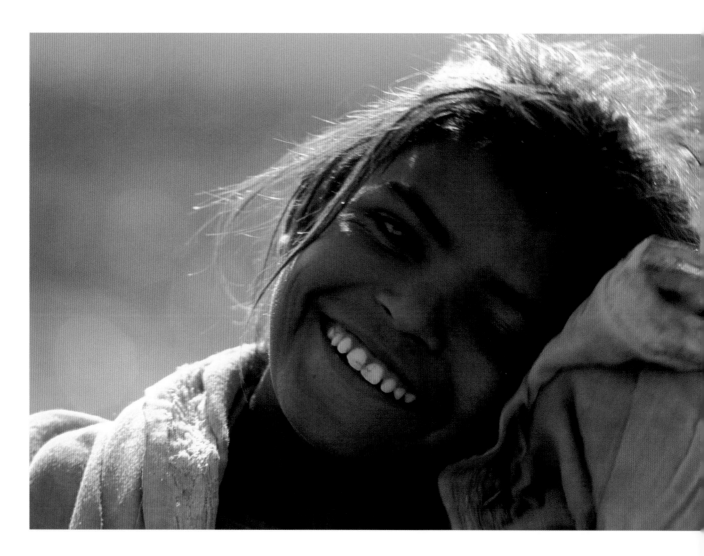

tobacco packaging raises awareness of the availability of quit line services (46), and the experience of several countries shows that it increases calls by smokers who are seeking assistance to quit (46).

Youth respond to warning labels

Youth respond to graphic health warning labels similarly to adults (16). Graphic warning labels are more likely to prevent adolescents from initiating smoking (47) or, if they are already smokers, to think about cutting down or quitting (48). Studies of children and adolescents find that mentioning specific diseases on health

warning labels makes them more believable than general warnings and that pictorial warnings are effective in making youth think about the health dangers of smoking and about reducing consumption (49–51).

Governments benefit from warning labels

Warning labels on tobacco packaging can be implemented at virtually no cost to government (28, 32). In general, warning labels are overwhelmingly supported by the public, often with levels of support at 85–90% or higher (52–54), and even most smokers support labelling requirements. Warnings also help gain public acceptance

of other tobacco control measures such as establishing smoke-free environments. It is important for national tobacco control programmes to monitor compliance with warning labelling requirements, as tobacco companies in some countries do not follow regulations even when enacted with force of law (55).

Health warnings in many countries can be made much stronger

Many countries, especially low- and middle-income countries, have health warning labels that are ineffective, and some do not mandate any warnings at all. In many

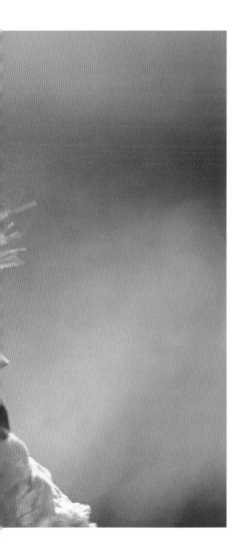

In general, warning labels are overwhelmingly supported by the public, often with levels of support at 85–90% or higher, and even most smokers support labelling requirements.

countries, warnings are weakly worded and vague, provide only general information without mention of specific health risks, and use small-sized print with no pictures. In some countries, warnings are not printed in a local language.

Some countries mandate stronger warning labels for manufactured cigarettes than for other tobacco products or for loose tobacco (56), which leads many people to believe that these products are less harmful (57). This is especially problematic in countries where there are high rates of use of local tobacco products other than manufactured cigarettes; these locally marketed products have typically not been covered by warning label requirements, and implementation of new labelling guidelines for them has been inconsistent.

Tobacco industry arguments against effective warning labels can be countered

The tobacco industry regularly fights implementation of health warnings because they are effective in changing attitudes about smoking (58), and the industry is especially resistant to large, graphic pictorial warnings (59). To prevent or delay implementation of health warnings, the tobacco industry makes various false claims, such as: people already know the risks of tobacco use; there is no evidence that pictorial warnings work; large, graphic health warnings violate tobacco company trademark and intellectual property rights; mandating warnings is too expensive; more time is needed to implement warnings; people who buy tobacco out of packaging (such as single cigarettes) will not see the warnings; graphic warnings demonize tobacco users;

Warning labels on tobacco packaging can be implemented at virtually no cost to government.

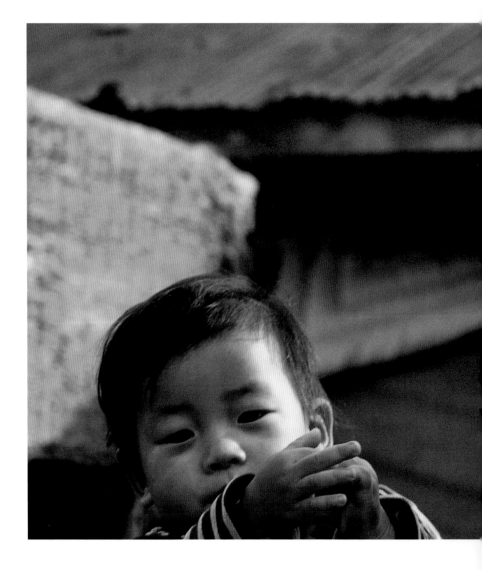

and governments should pay for their own advertising if they want to issue health warnings (60, 61). These false claims have often been used to attempt to block health warning legislation, but these spurious arguments can be countered with facts about the effectiveness and legality of warning labels. In Australia, some tobacco manufacturers have started including cards in cigarette packs that encourage smokers to complain to the government about the impending requirements for generic packaging and other tobacco control policies, including smoking bans and increased taxes (62).

WHO FCTC requirements and recommended guidelines on warning labels

Article 11 of the WHO FCTC requires that health warning labels on tobacco packaging conform to specified characteristics, including that they be approved by the competent national authority; cover at least 30% and preferably at least 50% of principal pack display areas; be large, clear, visible and legible and not use misleading terms (e.g. "light" or "mild"); be rotated either by using multiple warnings that appear concurrently or by introducing new warnings after a period of

time; display information on constituents and emissions of tobacco products; and appear in the principal language(s) of the country. The guidelines to Article 11 (2) include a number of other recommendations for health warning labels (see the previous chapter for full details of WHO FCTC warning label requirements and recommendations).

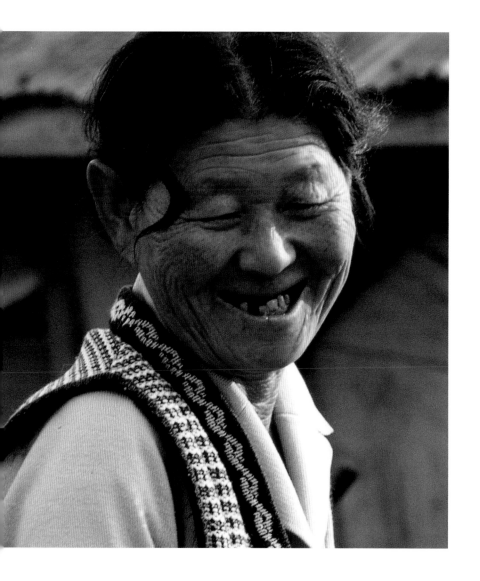

Warning labels that include pictures are most likely to be noticed and rated effective by smokers.

Anti-tobacco mass media campaigns

Media are important to tobacco control efforts

The media, which encompass journalistic reporting and commentary, entertainment programming and paid advertising and promotion, play a key role in shaping tobacco-related knowledge, opinions, attitudes and behaviours, and can be extremely powerful in influencing both individuals and policy-makers regarding tobacco use and tobacco control issues (16, 63, 64). As a result, mass media advertising campaigns have become a key component of tobacco control programmes (16, 65, 66).

In November 2010, the COP adopted guidelines for implementation of Article 12 of the WHO FCTC (Education, communication, training and public awareness) to assist Parties in meeting their treaty obligations (see the previous chapter for more details on Article 12 guidelines) (4).

Anti-tobacco mass media campaigns can reduce tobacco use

Anti-tobacco mass media campaigns are used to increase awareness of the harms of tobacco use and of second-hand smoke exposure, and in particular the harmful effects on health (67). Anti-tobacco advertising can also be used to explain the benefits of a tobacco-free society, or to reveal tobacco industry tactics that the public might find objectionable. Such campaigns contribute to changes in attitudes and beliefs of smokers that lead to changes in their smoking-related behaviour, specifically by reducing tobacco consumption and increasing motivation to make cessation attempts, as well as reducing exposure to second-hand smoke among non-smokers (16).

Anti-tobacco advertising sustains messaging about the dangers of tobacco. Advertising campaigns can be run in all types of media (television, radio, print, billboards and other outdoor display advertising, and online) (16), as well as on other items (e.g. matchbook covers) that are likely to be seen

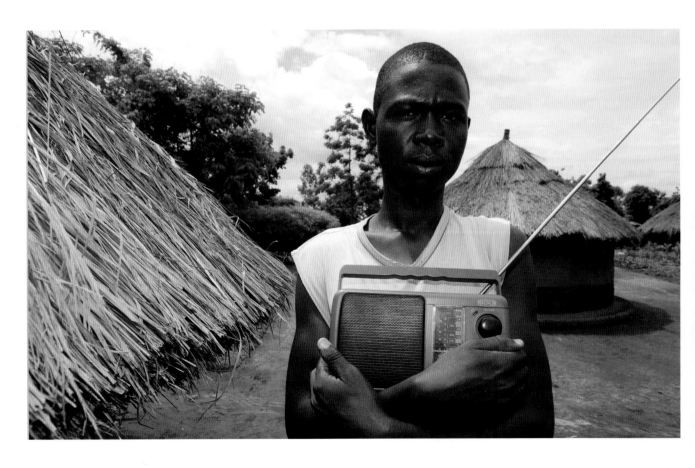

by smokers (*68*). Anti-tobacco mass media campaigns can be cost effective compared with other interventions despite the expense required (*69*), and can have a greater impact because they reach large populations quickly and efficiently (*16*).

Advertising can also help to counteract positive images of tobacco use portrayed by tobacco industry marketing and reverse the erroneous perception that tobacco use is a low-risk habit (*67*). Changing social norms about tobacco use in this way also increases support for other initiatives to reduce tobacco consumption (*70*).

A well-funded and intensive anti-tobacco mass media campaign is most effective as part of an ongoing, multi-faceted tobacco control programme, in part because synergies created by multiple interventions are capable of producing greater reductions in smoking than might be expected by merely adding together expected impacts of individual interventions (*16, 71, 72*). However, even in the absence of other tobacco control interventions, mass media campaigns have been shown to be effective on their own.

As is the case with health warning labels, most current evidence has examined the impact of mass media campaigns on cigarette smoking in high-income countries. However, evidence from low- and middle-income countries and for other types of tobacco use is growing (*73–75*).

Television is the most effective advertising medium

Television is generally considered to be the most powerful communications medium, and television advertising is especially effective (*16*). Anti-tobacco television advertising has higher recall than do advertisements in radio or print media (*76, 77*) because television facilitates the use of graphic imagery, which helps reinforce the association of tobacco with dangerous health consequences. These images more accurately depict the human impact of tobacco use by graphically showing suffering and illness, and can clearly portray tobacco use as socially undesirable and negative. In

Anti-tobacco mass media campaigns can be cost effective compared with other interventions despite the expense required, and can have a greater impact because they reach large populations quickly and efficiently.

countries where funding for anti-tobacco advertising campaigns is limited, use of less-expensive radio advertising may be an effective supplementary or alternative communications medium, especially in places where radio broadcasts reach a larger population than does television programming (78).

Exposure to effective anti-tobacco mass media campaigns has similar effects on adults and youth, with adult smokers more likely to quit (79) and youth less likely to become established smokers (80). Advertising campaigns broadcast at sufficient exposure levels and at frequent intervals reduce adult smoking prevalence (81, 82) and decrease youth smoking (83,

84); increase the numbers of smokers seeking cessation service from telephone quit lines (85) and increase adult cessation rates (86); result in steady positive changes in attitudes, beliefs and intentions to smoke among youth (87); and increase youth abstinence rates (88). Even limited exposure to anti-tobacco television advertising can increase intentions among youth not to smoke and reduce the likelihood of their becoming smokers in the future (89).

Results from GATS show that anti-tobacco advertisements on television and radio reach large segments of the population (90). Differences between countries may be related to the frequency and duration of existing anti-tobacco media campaigns, as

well as to differences in television and radio access.

Social media is increasing in importance

Although traditional media continue to have the widest population reach, use of the Internet and other emerging social media is expanding rapidly. These newer communications methods are becoming increasingly more effective in reaching youth, who in some cases are being exposed to them to a far greater extent than they are to other media. New media forms can be used to disseminate anti-smoking messages that prevent

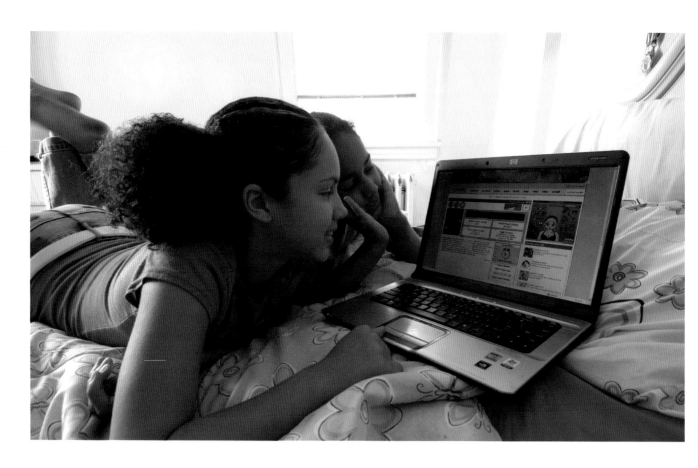

Campaigns using graphic images of illness and showing people suffering or dying demonstrate the harm caused by tobacco use, and are especially effective in convincing users to quit.

youth smoking initiation as well as assist adults with smoking cessation (*16, 91*). However, it is important that these emerging communications methods adhere to established evidence-based smoking cessation guidelines (e.g. counselling, quit lines and pharmacotherapy) (*92*).

Anti-tobacco mass media campaigns with hard-hitting themes help convince people to quit

Campaigns using graphic images of illness and showing people suffering or dying demonstrate the harm caused by

tobacco use, and are especially effective in convincing tobacco users to quit (*93–95*). Young and middle-aged adults should be the focus of advertisements whenever possible, whether they are suffering from tobacco-related illness themselves or are experiencing the negative effects of someone who is ill (e.g. A parent). This

HARD-HITTING ANTI-TOBACCO CAMPAIGNS ARE MORE EFFECTIVE THAN INFORMATIONAL CAMPAIGNS IN SÃO PAULO, BRAZIL

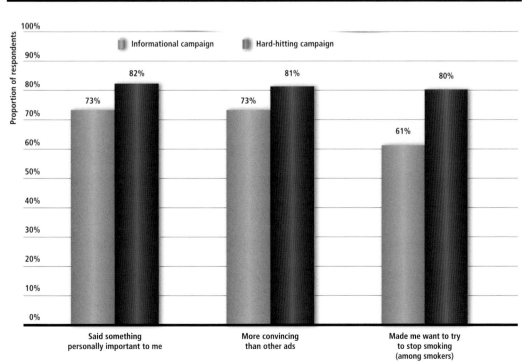

All differences shown are significant at $p<0.05$.
Source: (*74*).

Exposure to effective anti-tobacco mass media campaigns has similar effects on adults and youth, with adult smokers more likely to quit and youth less likely to become established smokers.

helps counteract widely held assumptions that only the elderly are affected by tobacco-related illness.

Campaigns developed primarily for adults can be equally effective among youth (96, 97), whereas advertising focused on youth does not have a similar impact on adults (98). Advertising that focuses on the health impact and other negative aspects of smoking appear to be the most effective among youth (16, 99–101), although

messages focusing on the harms of second-hand smoke and on tobacco industry deception are also promising strategies for preventing youth smoking (102, 103). Advertisements that make a strong emotional appeal are likely to increase recall among youth (104). Among adults, advertisements eliciting strong negative emotions are rated most effective, whereas humorous advertisements were seen as ineffective (16, 105). Among adult smokers who had recently quit, advertisements that

depict illness attributable to smoking or that provide practical advice on remaining tobacco-free are considered most helpful (106).

Anti-tobacco mass media campaigns are generally believed to be more effective when tailored to the cultural values of various targeted racial and ethnic groups, although this is not necessarily the case (107). At least among youth, content and other characteristics of advertisements

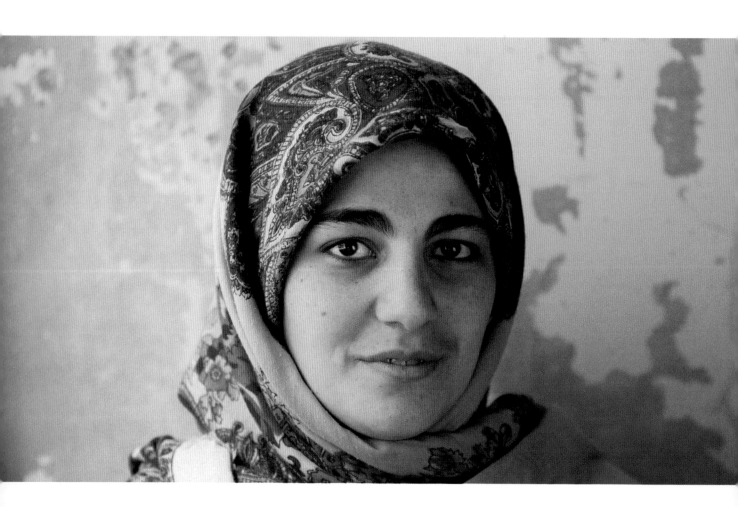

are more important than ethnicity or nationality in determining reactions to anti-tobacco advertising (108–110). Moreover, studies have shown that adult smokers and non-smokers alike react similarly to graphic images that induce an emotional response (105), despite perceived cultural or geographical differences. Use of message testing is important to ensure that the approaches chosen will resonate with target audiences.

Anti-tobacco mass media campaigns can promote smoking cessation services

Mass media advertising campaigns, which are an effective intervention in themselves, can also be a useful method for informing tobacco users about cessation services and directing them to quit lines (111). Promoting quit lines directly through advertising encourages smokers to seek assistance to quit (85). However, smoking cessation messages are most effective in an environment that aims to make smoking less socially acceptable.

In New York City, for example, which implements its own comprehensive municipal tobacco control programme, telephone calls for help to quit smoking quadrupled during a period of heavy anti-tobacco advertising compared with the same period the year before when there was no campaign (112). Studies also show that because people of lower socioeconomic status appear less responsive to anti-smoking television advertisements as measured by the rate of quit line calls, more needs to be done to reach disadvantaged groups (113).

Anti-tobacco mass media campaigns can be expensive, but are cost efficient

Although advertising campaigns can be a cost-efficient means of reaching large numbers of people, they can also be expensive, and television advertising is usually the most costly component of comprehensive tobacco control programmes (16). Countries can often successfully adapt advertising used elsewhere to save the time and expense needed to develop original campaign materials (114). This can be most easily done if there are no people

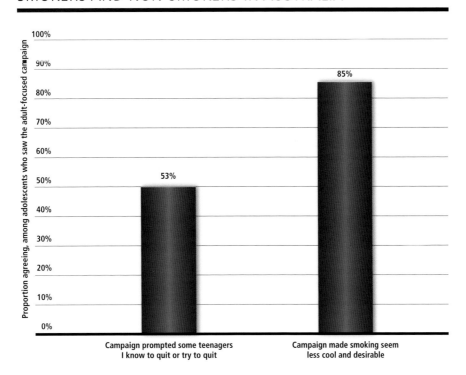

ADULT-FOCUSED CAMPAIGNS INFLUENCE ADOLESCENT SMOKERS AND NON-SMOKERS IN AUSTRALIA

Source: (97).

depicted in the campaign materials, but adaptation should also reflect differences in geographical context, racial and ethnic identity, and language. The priority should be on using or adapting existing materials that have already been evaluated for effectiveness. When no existing materials are appropriate, new ones should be pre-tested prior to widespread use whenever feasible.

In addition to the cost of broadcast air time and print media space, there are also production costs. Anti-tobacco advertisements should have the same production quality and persuasive power as tobacco industry advertising and marketing materials. Although production costs and air time or space must usually be paid for, they may also be provided free or at discount through government subsidies, funding from

nongovernmental organizations and grants of air time from broadcasters (16). Tobacco control programmes can also maximize the impact of their financial resources by, for example, pooling purchases with other government agencies to obtain larger volume discounts. Additionally, some governments allocate tobacco taxes or other government revenues to cover at least some of the costs of media campaigns.

In the 1960s in the United States, before tobacco advertising was banned on television, television broadcasters were required to run free anti-tobacco advertisements; these were effective in reducing tobacco consumption, smoking prevalence and smoking initiation (115–117). Currently, some countries mandate that broadcasters provide free air time for anti-tobacco television advertising

campaigns, though the quantity and content of such advertising varies widely.

According to studies, governments in high-income countries should spend about US$ 1.50–4.00 per person per year on anti-tobacco health communication and counter-advertising (about 15–20% of total tobacco control expenditures) (70). However, there is currently a lack of comparable estimates and recommendations for low- and middle-income countries.

Anti-tobacco mass media campaigns need to be sustained

Because the effects of advertising are often complex and indirectly diffused through other interventions (118), anti-tobacco

ANTI-TOBACCO MASS MEDIA CAMPAIGNS INCREASE CALLS FOR CESSATION ASSISTANCE IN VICTORIA, AUSTRALIA

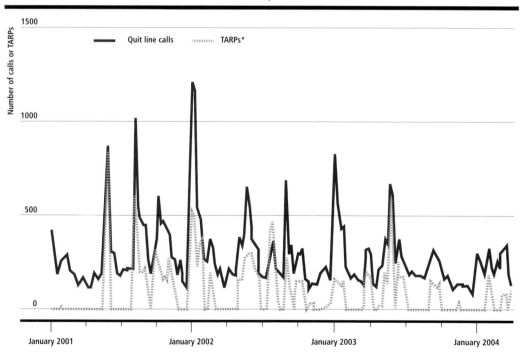

* Television Advertising Rating Points (TARPs) are a standard measure of television advertising weight and are used to indicate the number of people within a certain demographic group that were exposed to an advertisement within a given period of time.
Source: (113).

advertising strategies generally require sustained exposure over long periods to have a lasting effect (119). Advertising campaigns should run at least six months to effect awareness of issues, 12–18 months to have an impact on attitudes, and 18–24 months to change behaviour (120). The longer an anti-tobacco media campaign is established, the more likely it will result in sustained declines in both adult and youth smoking (79, 81, 121). However, because many tobacco control programmes are unlikely to have sufficient resources to run campaigns of this duration, and because shorter-term campaigns can have some impact, these recommendations should be considered as a goal and should not dissuade campaigns of shorter duration.

Conversely, suspension of anti-tobacco advertising campaigns may increase

smoking (122–124). Campaigns lasting as little as three weeks may have a measurable impact in reducing smoking uptake among youth, especially if they use provocative themes, are repeated in successive years, and are augmented with advertising in print and other media (125). Television advertisements that are emotionally arousing require fewer broadcasts than less engaging messages to achieve viewer recall, which can decrease the costs of a campaign (104).

Planning and evaluation are important campaign components

Ongoing planning and evaluation are necessary to develop anti-tobacco advertising campaigns and assess their

effectiveness. As with any type of social marketing project, the process must include planning, implementation and evaluation phases. The table below outlines the steps to be taken in each phase and the performance objectives for each campaign component (126).

The tobacco industry fights to stop anti-tobacco mass media campaigns

As part of its strategy to weaken tobacco control efforts generally, the tobacco industry typically works to prevent or limit the effectiveness of anti-tobacco advertising campaigns, often claiming that they are inaccurate and a misuse of government resources (16). Ensuring that all anti-tobacco mass media campaigns are based

FRAMEWORK FOR THE DEVELOPMENT OF AN ANTI-TOBACCO MASS MEDIA CAMPAIGN

Phase	Assessment domain	Performance objective
Planning Identification of target audiences; planning of objectives, strategies and activities; and adaptation or development of materials	Tobacco control strategy	Campaign is integral component of comprehensive tobacco control programme
	Formative research	Thorough understanding of target audience knowledge, attitudes and smoking behaviour is gained to guide objectives and strategies
	Pre-testing	Materials pre-tested and refined to meet campaign objectives
Implementation Design and implementation of media strategy to maximize target audience exposures and impact	Advertising placement	Media planning and buying effectively and efficiently reaches campaign target audience
	Earned media and public relations	Additional unpaid media coverage for the campaign is gained
Evaluation Assessment of campaign implementation and impact	Process evaluation	Assess campaign implementation
	Outcome evaluation	Assess campaign impact

Source: (126).

on statements that are easily verifiable by scientific evidence will help to withstand this type of challenge. The tobacco industry has created its own anti-tobacco advertising, often in response to government actions to curtail its business practices, to avoid even more restrictive future regulation and to try to promote its image as a good corporate citizen (16, 127, 128). However, these efforts are often thinly disguised product advertisements (16), are ineffective in reducing smoking, and may even increase smoking, especially among youth (87,101,129–132). The guidelines to WHO FCTC Article 5.3 (133) include a number of recommendations to prevent government agencies from partnering with the tobacco industry in the implementation of youth smoking prevention and other campaigns.

"Earned" media can have a large impact

The process of obtaining media exposure without spending money on paid advertising is known as "earned" media, reflecting that the coverage is earned through public relations efforts instead of being paid for. The news media represent a key source of health information for the general public as well as a framing mechanism for the overall tobacco control agenda, which itself has become increasingly more newsworthy (16). Tobacco control efforts can be supplemented through media advocacy efforts, although this approach is often underused (16). Obtaining free news coverage can be a highly effective and inexpensive way to inform the public

about the harms of tobacco, gain attention for tobacco control initiatives, and counter tobacco industry misinformation (134).

Media outreach efforts should be proactive and engage the media whenever there are developments in tobacco control. Because the media often wish to be seen as advocates for the public good (135) and are likely to report favourably on tobacco control issues (16), it is important to ensure that any news stories contain a strong tobacco control advocacy viewpoint. At a minimum, issuing press releases can sometimes result in substantial media coverage (136).

Increased news coverage of tobacco control issues may reduce tobacco consumption and

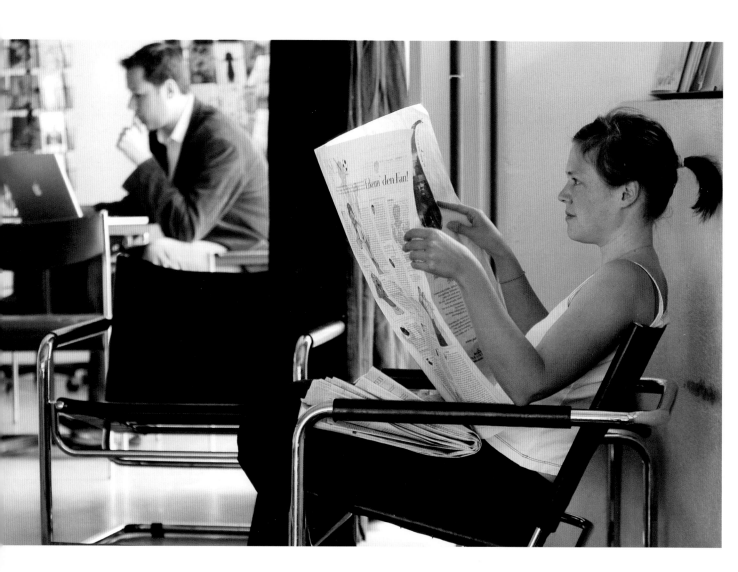

increase cessation attempts (*137–139*) and, among youth, increases the perceptions of harm caused by smoking (*140*). Well-managed publicity supporting mass media campaigns can have a large impact on the number of people aware of and responding to a campaign. Earned media can also be effective in motivating smokers to quit when tobacco control policy changes are put into effect (*141*).

WHO FCTC requirements and guidelines on education, communication, training and public awareness

Article 12 of the WHO FCTC requires Parties to promote and strengthen public awareness of tobacco control issues, using all available communication tools, as appropriate. Towards this end, Parties are obligated to promote educational programmes on the health risks of tobacco use and exposure to tobacco smoke and about the benefits of cessation. They should also provide the public with access to information about the tobacco industry and about the adverse health, economic and environmental consequences of tobacco production and consumption. Awareness programmes addressed to health workers, community workers, educators, decision-makers and other concerned persons are also to be promoted. Parties are further obligated to foster the development of intersectoral programmes among public and private agencies and NGOs. The

guidelines to Article 12 (*4*) include a number of other recommendations for education, communication, training and public awareness (see the previous chapter for full details of recommendations).

Obtaining free news coverage can be a highly effective and inexpensive way to inform the public about the harms of tobacco, gain attention for tobacco control initiatives, and counter tobacco industry misinformation.

Implementation of effective measures continues to gain momentum

Monitor tobacco use and prevention policies

The WHO Framework Convention on Tobacco Control states (1): Article 20: … Parties shall establish … surveillance of the magnitude, patterns, determinants and consequences of tobacco consumption and exposure to tobacco smoke … Parties should integrate tobacco surveillance programmes into national, regional and global health surveillance programmes so that data are comparable and can be analysed at the regional and international levels … Article 21: Each Party shall submit … periodic reports on its implementation of this Convention …

RECENT ACHIEVEMENTS AND DEVELOPMENTS

By the end of 2010, the Global Adult Tobacco Survey (GATS) was completed in 14 low- and middle-income countries, representing 54% of the world's population. All GATS data are internationally comparable and provide rigorous estimates of tobacco use. GATS also tracks the progress of MPOWER measures as well as gaps in policy development. Tobacco Questions for Surveys (TQS), a short set of standardized questions that measure tobacco use and progress of the MPOWER measures, will be released in 2011. These questions are consistent with those used in GATS and can be used by countries in an existing or planned survey to assure tobacco prevalence results that are internationally comparable.

PREVALENCE OF ADULT TOBACCO USE IN THE 14 COUNTRIES THAT COMPLETED THE GLOBAL ADULT TOBACCO SURVEY, 2008–2010

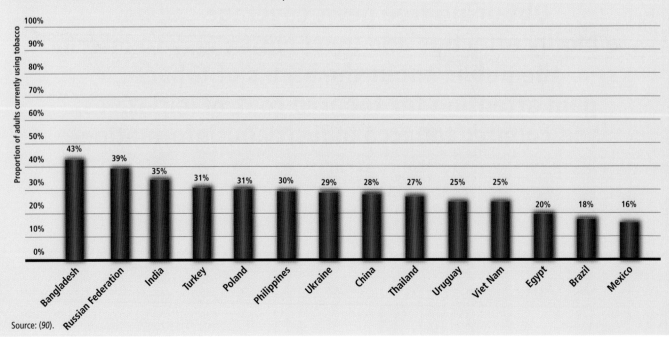

Source: (90).

MONITORING

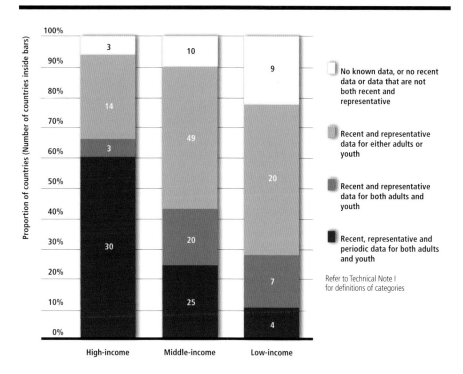

Monitoring of tobacco use and tobacco control policy achievements is critical to understanding and reversing the epidemic and ensuring success of the other five MPOWER measures.

MONITOR THE PREVALENCE OF TOBACCO USE – HIGHEST ACHIEVING COUNTRIES, 2010

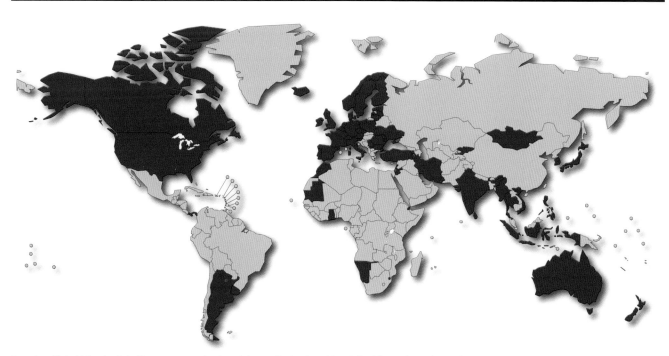

Countries with the highest level of achievement: Argentina, Armenia*, Australia, Austria, Belgium, Bulgaria*, Canada, Czech Republic, Denmark, Djibouti*, Estonia, Finland, France, Germany, Ghana*, Iceland*, India, Indonesia*, Iran (Islamic Republic of), Ireland, Israel, Italy, Japan, Jordan, Kyrgyzstan*, Latvia, Lebanon*, Lithuania, Luxembourg*, Malta, Mauritania, Mongolia*, Morocco*, Myanmar*, Namibia*, Netherlands, New Zealand*, Norway, Panama*, Philippines*, Poland, Portugal, Republic of Korea, Republic of Moldova*, Romania*, Serbia, Slovenia, Spain, Sri Lanka*, Swaziland, Sweden, Switzerland, Thailand*, Turkey*, Ukraine*, United Kingdom of Great Britain and Northern Ireland, United States of America, Uruguay and Viet Nam*

* Country newly at the highest level since 31 December 2008.

Monitoring is critical to tobacco control efforts

Monitoring of tobacco use and tobacco control policy achievements is critical to understanding and reversing the epidemic and ensuring success of the other five MPOWER measures (*142*). Good monitoring systems should track indicators of tobacco use, including use of smokeless tobacco and new, emerging forms of tobacco (water pipe, e-cigarettes), as well as the impact of policy interventions (*143*). Tobacco industry activities should also be monitored (*14*). Accurate data allow for appropriate policy implementation, efficient impact measurement and timely adjustment when necessary, all which greatly improve the likelihood of success (*14*).

Tobacco use monitoring has been strengthened in some countries, but remains weak in many others

Since publication of the *WHO Report on the Global Tobacco Epidemic, 2009*, there are 23 additional countries that have strengthened tobacco use monitoring to include recent and representative data for both adults and youth, and have also conducted ongoing periodic surveys that collect these data at least every five years. The total number of countries reporting this level of monitoring practice is 59, representing about 3.2 billion people, or almost half of the world's population.

Despite this significant progress, more than 100 countries still do not have representative data for both adults and youth, or have no data at all – and an additional 30 countries do not have periodic data, making it difficult to accurately track trends in tobacco use. GATS, introduced in 14 countries during 2009 and 2010, is an important tool that has strengthened monitoring in a number of countries and can serve as a model for conducting high-quality monitoring. It is important that countries develop and conduct surveys on tobacco use and tobacco control policy implementation, either as part of general health surveys or as stand-alone tobacco surveys, to provide the data needed to effectively fight the global tobacco epidemic.

It is important that countries develop and conduct surveys on tobacco use and tobacco control policy implementation, either as part of general health surveys or as stand-alone tobacco surveys.

Philippines implements GATS and other tobacco use surveys

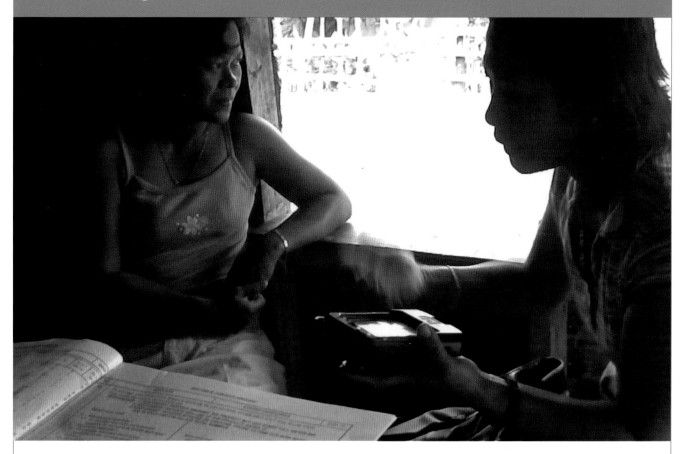

The Philippines has a strong and well-developed health surveillance infrastructure. Monitoring of tobacco use and its determinants has been conducted in the Philippines since 1989 under the leadership of the Department of Health. Numerous surveys have been administered by various agencies at national and subnational levels, including a National Nutrition and Health Survey using the WHO-STEPS survey instrument.

This report shows that the Philippines' tobacco use monitoring system includes periodic, recent and representative smoking prevalence data for both adults and youth, ranking the country in the highest category of monitoring effectiveness.

Among youth, the Global Youth Tobacco Survey (GYTS) was conducted in 2000, 2004 and 2007. The GYTS surveys students in their second, third and fourth years of secondary school, and yields representative estimates of smoking prevalence among students aged 13–15 years. The 2000 survey showed that 31% of boys and 18% of girls were current tobacco users. After declines to 21% among boys and to 12% among girls in 2004, the 2007 survey showed a resurgence in tobacco use to 28% for boys and 18% for girls (*144*).

Additionally, the Global Health Professions Student Survey was conducted in 2005 among students in their third year of pharmacy school, and in 2009 among students in the third year of medical school. The 2005 survey showed that 38% of male and 18% of female pharmacy students were current smokers; that more than half of students who had never smoked were regularly exposed to second-hand tobacco smoke at home and more than three quarters were exposed in public places; and that nearly 90% of pharmacy students believed that all enclosed public spaces should be completely smoke-free (*145*).

The most recent measure of tobacco use in the Philippines, GATS, was conducted in 2009. A total of 9705 adults were interviewed, producing a nationally representative sample of the adult household population 15 years of age and older. The survey showed that 48% of men and 9% of women are current smokers; that in the month prior to the survey 37% of adults had been exposed to second-hand tobacco smoke at workplaces and 54% had been exposed at home; and that more people noticed anti-tobacco information in the media (80%) than noticed advertisements for cigarettes (71%) (*146*).

mpower Protect from tobacco smoke

The WHO Framework Convention on Tobacco Control states (1): Article 8: … scientific evidence has unequivocally established that exposure to tobacco smoke causes death, disease and disability … [Parties] shall adopt and implement … measures providing for protection from exposure to tobacco smoke in indoor workplaces, public transport, indoor public places and, as appropriate, other public places. WHO FCTC Article 8 guidelines (147) are intended to assist Parties in meeting their obligations under Article 8 of the Convention and provide a clear timeline for Parties to adopt appropriate measures (within five years after entry into Force of the WHO FCTC).

Second-hand smoke kills

There is no safe level of exposure to second-hand smoke, which contributes to a range of serious and often fatal diseases, including heart disease, respiratory illness, and lung and other cancers (148). Children can also be harmed by second-hand smoke exposure, and babies in utero and newborns are particularly susceptible (148).

Smoke-free laws save lives

Completely smoke-free environments with no exceptions are the only proven way to protect people from second-hand smoke (148). Separate smoking rooms and ventilation systems do not prevent second-hand smoke exposure (148). Governments must maintain strong support for laws once they are enacted through proactive and uniform enforcement that achieves high compliance levels (148).

Experience in a growing number of countries and subnational areas shows that it is possible to enact and enforce effective smoke-free laws, and that doing so is popular with the public, does not harm business, and improves health (149). Public opinion polling continues to show consistent strong support for smoke-free laws wherever they are enacted (148). Smoke-free environments also help smokers who want to quit, and encourage people to make their homes smoke-free to protect children and other non-smokers (148).

Smoke-free laws do not hurt business

Despite tobacco and hospitality industry claims, experience shows that in every country where comprehensive smoke-free legislation has been enacted, smoke-free environments are popular, easy to implement and enforce, and result in either

SMOKE-FREE LEGISLATION

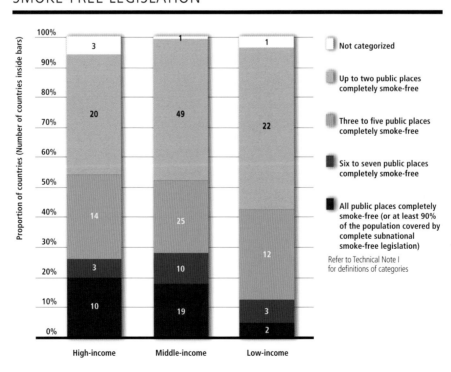

RECENT ACHIEVEMENTS AND DEVELOPMENTS

Results from GATS show that large numbers of people continue to be exposed to second-hand tobacco smoke at home and in the workplace. Exposure to second-hand smoke is lower in countries with comprehensive smoke-free laws than in countries with smoking bans covering only some types of public places or none at all.

The 2010 United States Surgeon General's report contains new scientific data that confirm the health harms caused by tobacco smoke, and detail the biological and behavioural mechanisms of how mainstream and second-hand smoke damage the human body (*150*). The evidence and conclusions in this report validate earlier findings, expand and strengthen the science base, and describe in great detail the multiple ways that even small levels of exposure to tobacco smoke damage every organ in the body, resulting in disease and death.

Study results published by the United States Institute of Medicine consistently indicate that second-hand smoke exposure increases the risk of coronary heart disease by 25–30% in non-smokers, and that there are increased risks even at the lowest levels of exposure (*151*). Studies show a 6–47% decrease in the rate of heart attacks in smokers and non-smokers after smoking bans are implemented (*151*).

NON-SMOKING ADULTS WORKING INDOORS WHO ARE EXPOSED TO SECOND-HAND TOBACCO SMOKE IN THE WORKPLACE IN THE 14 COUNTRIES THAT COMPLETED GATS, 2008–2010

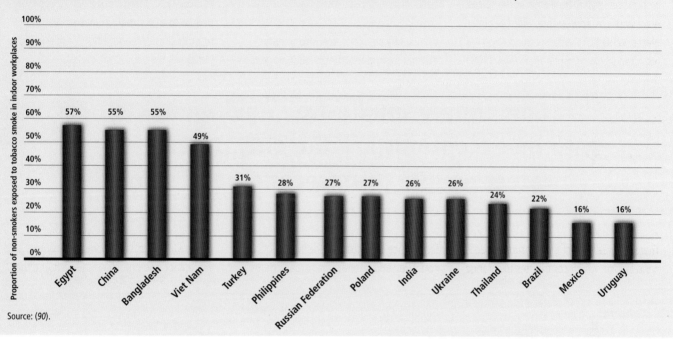

Source: (*90*).

SMOKE-FREE ENVIRONMENTS – HIGHEST ACHIEVING COUNTRIES, 2010

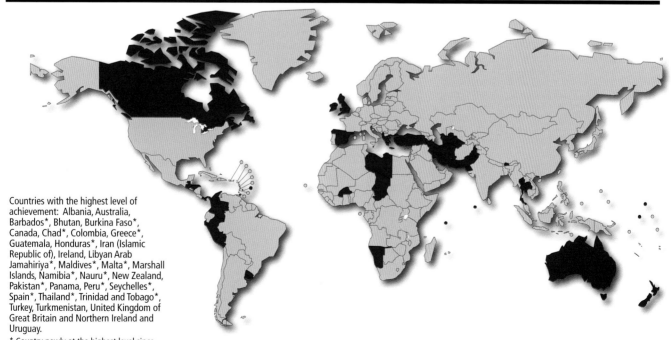

Countries with the highest level of achievement: Albania, Australia, Barbados*, Bhutan, Burkina Faso*, Canada, Chad*, Colombia, Greece*, Guatemala, Honduras*, Iran (Islamic Republic of), Ireland, Libyan Arab Jamahiriya*, Maldives*, Malta*, Marshall Islands, Namibia*, Nauru*, New Zealand, Pakistan*, Panama, Peru*, Seychelles*, Spain*, Thailand*, Trinidad and Tobago*, Turkey, Turkmenistan, United Kingdom of Great Britain and Northern Ireland and Uruguay.

* Country newly at the highest level since 31 December 2008.

a neutral or positive impact on businesses, including the hospitality sector (*149*).

Notable progress has been achieved in enacting smoke-free policies

Between 2008 and 2010, 16 countries newly enacted nationwide comprehensive smoke-free legislation, increasing to 31 the number of countries that provide the highest level of protection against second-hand tobacco smoke exposure. More than 739 million people, representing almost 11% of the world's population, are protected by comprehensive, national smoke-free laws, an increase of more than 385 million since 2008.

Middle-income countries were especially active in expanding these protections through enacting smoke-free laws that cover all or some types of public places (see Technical Note I). About half of countries in each income classification have legislation covering more than two types of public places, but the other half still have only minimal policies with legislation covering only one or two types of public places, or have no laws at all.

An additional 210 million people (3% of the world's population) are protected by comprehensive smoke-free legislation at the subnational level, an increase of almost 100 million since 2008. Notable gains were made in Brazil, which now protects 77 million people (representing nearly 40% of its population) by subnational smoke-free laws passed since 2008, and in the United States, which now protects 21 million more people at the subnational level.

Completely smoke-free environments with no exceptions are the only proven way to protect people from second-hand smoke.

DISEASES CAUSED BY SMOKING AND EXPOSURE TO SECOND-HAND SMOKE

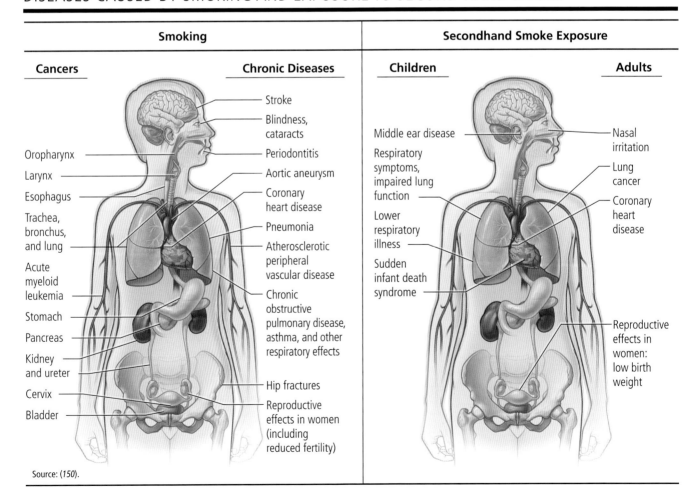

Source: (*150*).

Passage of a strong smoke-free law in the Seychelles caps long-term tobacco control efforts

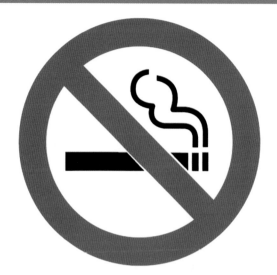

DEFANN FIMEN

I KONT LALWA POU FIMEN DAN SA LANDRWA

"Smoking is forbidden; it is against the law to smoke in these premises."

In the Seychelles, located in an archipelago in the Indian Ocean, strong progress has been made on several WHO FCTC Articles, including Article 8 (Protection from exposure to tobacco smoke).

The country's Tobacco Control Act of August 2009 created completely smoke-free environments in all enclosed public places and workplaces, on all transport, and in selected outdoor premises including all health and educational facilities and all stadiums. Tobacco advertising, promotion and sponsorship are also completely banned, formalizing the absence of tobacco advertising that has been observed for several decades and extending it to new forms of tobacco marketing.

Data collected for this report show that the Act has been unanimously assessed as having high compliance by tobacco control experts. A recent survey also showed good compliance with the law; compliance was checked in 38 of the country's most popular hospitality venues and in 97% of these premises no customers were seen smoking (152).

Comprehensive tobacco control legislation was first drafted in the Seychelles in 1996, but not enacted. A national committee for tobacco control, established in 2000 by the Minister of Health, elaborated a new draft of comprehensive legislation that was rejected several times primarily because of the total ban on smoking in enclosed public places. With the assistance of international tobacco control experts, communities mobilized to support the legislation, and advocated in particular for the smoke-free regulations. This advocacy was key to the law being passed in June 2009 by unanimous vote in the National Assembly. Passage of the Act also continues the Seychelles tradition of being in the forefront of tobacco control, including being the first country in the African Region to ratify the WHO FCTC in 2003, and may serve as a model for other countries.

More than 739 million people are protected by comprehensive, national smoke-free laws, an increase of more than 385 million since 2008.

mpower Offer help to quit tobacco use

The WHO Framework Convention on Tobacco Control states (1): Article 14: Each Party shall … take effective measures to promote cessation of tobacco use and adequate treatment for tobacco dependence … Each Party shall … design and implement effective programmes aimed at promoting the cessation of tobacco use. WHO FCTC Article 14 guidelines (153) are intended to assist Parties in meeting their obligations under Article 14 of the Convention.

Most smokers want to quit

Most smokers who are aware of the dangers of tobacco want to quit, but quitting without assistance is difficult because nicotine is highly addictive

(143). Although most who quit eventually do so without intervention, assistance greatly increases quit rates (143). Quitting produces immediate and significant health benefits and reduces most of the associated risks within a few years of quitting (143).

Tobacco cessation interventions are effective

Clinical cessation interventions are extremely cost-effective compared with other health-care system activities (14). Three types of treatment should be included in any tobacco prevention effort (143).

- Cessation advice in health care. Brief advice from primary health-care

practitioners increases quit rates (143).
- Quit lines. Cessation advice and counselling can also be provided in the form of free telephone help lines (known as quit lines) (143).
- Pharmacological therapy. Cessation can also include treatment with nicotine replacement therapy (NRT), usually available over the counter, and other drugs that require a prescription (143). Pharmacological therapy can double or triple quit rates (143, 154).

Government support for cessation treatment

Smoking cessation is primarily the responsibility of each country's health-care system (143). Cessation services are

TOBACCO DEPENDENCE TREATMENT

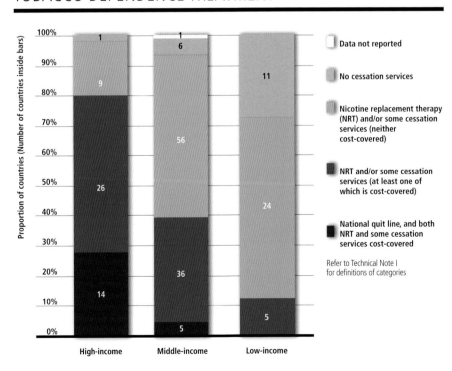

RECENT ACHIEVEMENTS AND DEVELOPMENTS

In November 2010, the fourth session of the COP to the WHO FCTC issued detailed guidelines for implementation of Article 14 (Demand reduction measures concerning tobacco dependence and cessation) (153). These guidelines are intended to encourage Parties to strengthen or create a sustainable infrastructure to motivate quit attempts and ensure wide access to cessation support and dependence treatment, identify key effective measures to promote cessation and incorporate treatment into national tobacco control programmes and health-care systems, and urge Parties to share experiences and collaborate in order to facilitate development or strengthening of support for cessation and treatment.

To better meet countries' anticipated need for technical support to scale up treatment and cessation capacity, the WHO TFI has developed a comprehensive training package, *Strengthening Primary Health Care (PHC) Systems for Treating Tobacco Dependence*, to assist countries in implementing Article 14 of the WHO FCTC and strengthening their primary health-care systems for treating tobacco dependence. The training package has been piloted in five countries (Bahamas, Barbados, Iran, Panama, and Trinidad and Tobago) and will be finalized and disseminated in 2011 after additional pilot tests in two more countries.

ADULT SMOKERS PLANNING TO QUIT OR THINKING ABOUT QUITTING SMOKING IN THE 14 COUNTRIES THAT COMPLETED GATS, 2008–2010

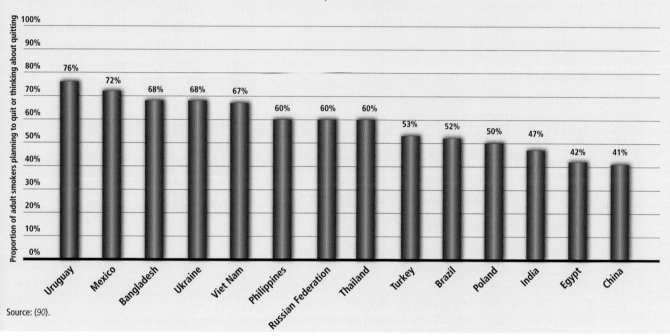

Source: (90).

TOBACCO DEPENDENCE TREATMENT – HIGHEST ACHIEVING COUNTRIES, 2010

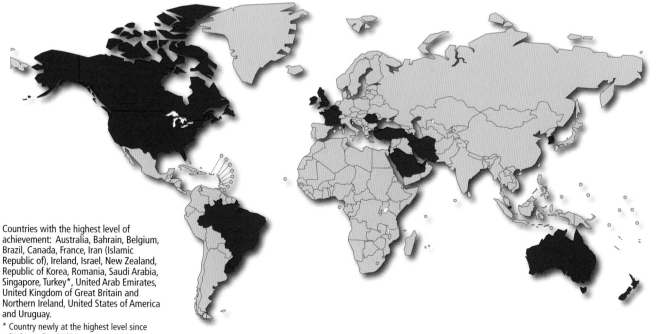

Countries with the highest level of achievement: Australia, Bahrain, Belgium, Brazil, Canada, France, Iran (Islamic Republic of), Ireland, Israel, New Zealand, Republic of Korea, Romania, Saudi Arabia, Singapore, Turkey*, United Arab Emirates, United Kingdom of Great Britain and Northern Ireland, United States of America and Uruguay.

* Country newly at the highest level since 31 December 2008.

most effective when they are part of a coordinated tobacco control programme (143).

Minimal progress has been made in providing access to comprehensive help to quit smoking

Between 2008 and 2010, one additional country (Turkey) began providing comprehensive[1] tobacco dependence treatment that includes a national quit line as well as coverage of costs for nicotine replacement therapy and at least some other cessation services. This brings the number of countries that provide the highest level of tobacco cessation services to 19, which now cover 980 million people (about 14% of the world's population), an increase of 76 million since 2008.

High-income countries, which are expected to have the necessary financial resources, were most likely to provide and fund a full range of cessation services, although less than 30% of countries in this income classification currently do so. Both high- and middle-income countries showed progress in providing at least some cost coverage for tobacco dependence treatment, with 80% of high-income and nearly 40% of middle-income countries now providing services at this level or greater. However, no low-income country yet offers a national quit line as well as cost-covered cessation services, and only one in eight currently covers any costs of cessation services.

[1] "Comprehensive" refers to countries qualifying for the top group of the O indicator; see Technical Note I for details.

Quitting produces immediate and significant health benefits and reduces most of the associated risks within a few years of quitting.

SMOKERS REPORTING SIX MONTHS' CONTINUED CESSATION WITH DIFFERENT INTERVENTIONS

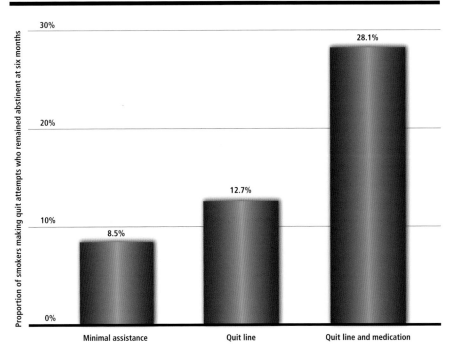

Source: (154).

New Zealand offers comprehensive no-cost cessation services

New Zealand (*Aotearoa*) provides a wide range of free cessation services as part of its comprehensive tobacco control strategy. Smoking prevalence among adults in 2009 was 21%, a decline by about a third over the past two decades that resulted from sustained strong tobacco control policies and high-quality cessation services. New Zealand first introduced nationally funded cessation programmes in the late 1990s: a national quit line service, based on established international models, and *Aukati Kaipaipa*, a programme targeted to the indigenous Maori population.

The national quit line (http://www.quit.org.nz) now assists more than 50 000 New Zealanders each year who attempt to quit smoking. It has also expanded to include text messaging and online services, with a blog community of over 30 000 members who share cessation experiences and offer tips, support and encouragement to help others towards a smoke-free future.

Aukati Kaipaipa's services, which have similarly grown from an initial pilot to more than 30 sites throughout the country, feature professional Quit Coaches who deliver face-to-face services "to Maori, by Maori". Personalized counselling programmes include intensive support for the initial 12 weeks, with follow-up every three months for the first year. This model has been highly effective for many people who might not have sought out less personalized models of support.

In the same period, ensuring "better help for smokers to quit" was given formal status as one of only six governmental priority health targets – with an ultimate goal that 90% of all smokers who enter New Zealand hospitals receive advice and assistance to quit. New Zealand's health system uses an ABC approach: **Ask** smoking status, give **Brief** advice, offer **Cessation** support. As of May 2011, since the Health Target was first introduced in 2009, over 110 000 have received brief advice to quit smoking in the hospital setting alone.

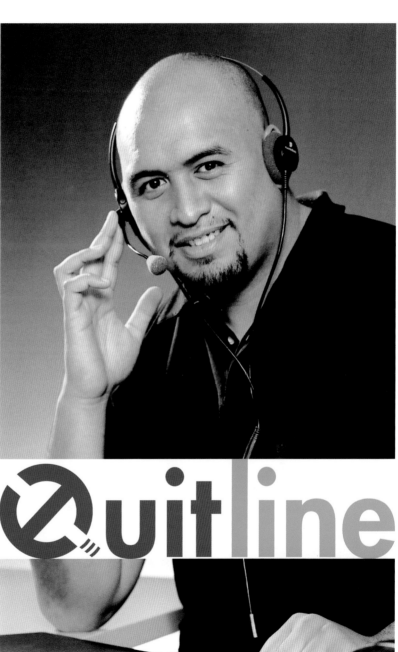

mpower

Health warning labels

The number of people exposed to strong graphic health warning labels on tobacco packaging has almost doubled

Three additional countries (Mexico, Peru and the United States) passed new laws between 2008 and 2010 that strengthened requirements for health warning labels on tobacco products so that they cover at least 50% of principal pack display areas and include all major characteristics outlined in WHO FCTC Article 11, including the use of pictures. A total of 19 countries with more than 1 billion people (almost 15% of the world's population) now mandate health warning labels at this level of best practice, an increase from 10 countries in 2007 and 16 countries in 2008. This nearly doubles

the number of people worldwide who have been newly exposed to strong graphic health warnings since 2008, when 8% of the world's population was protected, and almost triples the coverage of this intervention at this highest level since 2007, when 5% of the world's population was covered.

People in high- and middle-income countries are more likely to be protected by strong warning labels

High- and middle-income countries had the only increases in populations covered by best-practice warning labels. The number of middle-income countries with strong warning labels at the best-practice level has doubled since 2007. Since 2008, four low-income

countries have made some progress in strengthening warning labels, but no country in this income category has yet reached the best-practice level. There are 87 countries in all income classifications that mandate only small warnings covering less than 30% of pack surface areas or that have no requirements at all for warning labels, with low-income countries particularly likely to have weak warning label requirements.

Most countries mandate at least some labelling, but many have not yet implemented best-practice warning labels

Of the cigarette pack warning label characteristics assessed for the reporting

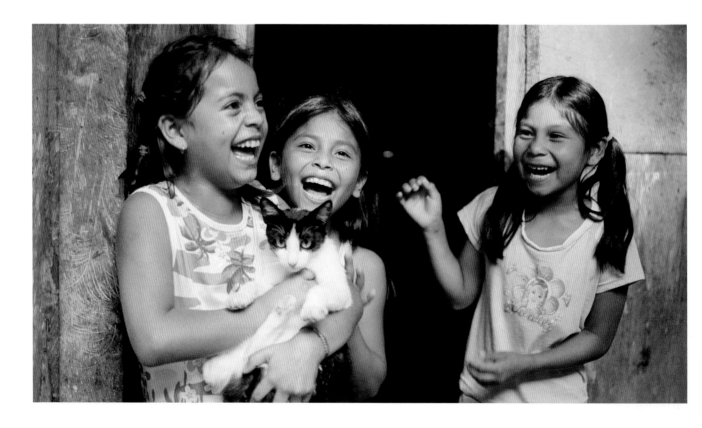

WARNING LABELS

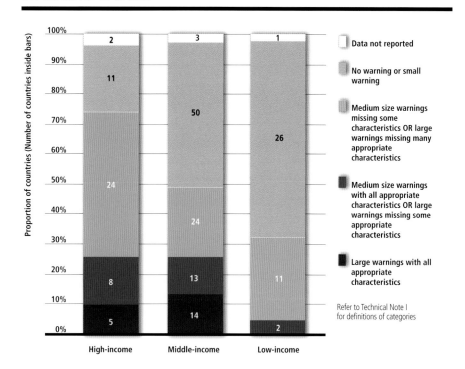

Proportion of countries (Number of countries inside bars)

High-income: 2, 11, 24, 8, 5
Middle-income: 3, 50, 24, 13, 14
Low-income: 1, 26, 11, 2

Legend:
- Data not reported
- No warning or small warning
- Medium size warnings missing some characteristics OR large warnings missing many appropriate characteristics
- Medium size warnings with all appropriate characteristics OR large warnings missing some appropriate characteristics
- Large warnings with all appropriate characteristics

Refer to Technical Note I for definitions of categories

Health warning labels that are large and incorporate pictorial images reduce tobacco consumption and save lives.

HEALTH WARNING LABELS ABOUT THE DANGERS OF TOBACCO – HIGHEST ACHIEVING COUNTRIES, 2010

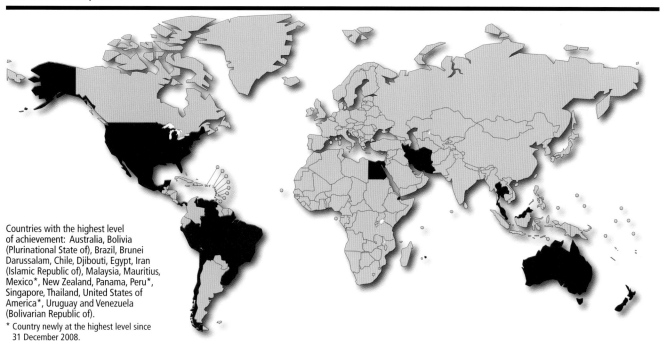

Countries with the highest level of achievement: Australia, Bolivia (Plurinational State of), Brazil, Brunei Darussalam, Chile, Djibouti, Egypt, Iran (Islamic Republic of), Malaysia, Mauritius, Mexico*, New Zealand, Panama, Peru*, Singapore, Thailand, United States of America*, Uruguay and Venezuela (Bolivarian Republic of).

* Country newly at the highest level since 31 December 2008.

categories in this report, the most frequently legislated are mandating specific health warnings and having warnings that appear on each individual package as well as on outside packaging (e.g. carton wrappers). In both cases, 130 countries had warnings with these characteristics.

The least frequently legislated characteristic is the requirement for a large warning label size, with only 30 countries mandating pack warnings that cover 50% or more of main pack display areas (i.e. the front and back of the packs). The second least legislated

characteristic is warnings that feature a photograph or other pictorial graphic, which was adopted by only 42 countries.

Health warning labels that are large in size and that incorporate pictorial images provide the most effective types of warnings; implementing these characteristics more widely would reduce tobacco consumption and save lives.

Other warning label characteristics legislated by half or less of all countries are requirements that labels be printed using

specified font styles, sizes and colours to ensure easy legibility, as well as periodic rotation of warning labels so that they stay fresh in people's minds and continue to have an impact.

Although not included in the determination of best practice for this report, banning misleading descriptive terms, such as "light" and "mild", is also important because these descriptors may give the false impression that some tobacco products are less harmful than others. In total, 89 countries ban these misleading terms for manufactured

A total of 19 countries with more than 1 billion people now mandate best-practice health warning labels.

HEALTH WARNINGS ON CIGARETTE PACKAGING, NUMBER OF COUNTRIES LEGISLATING EACH CHARACTERISTIC

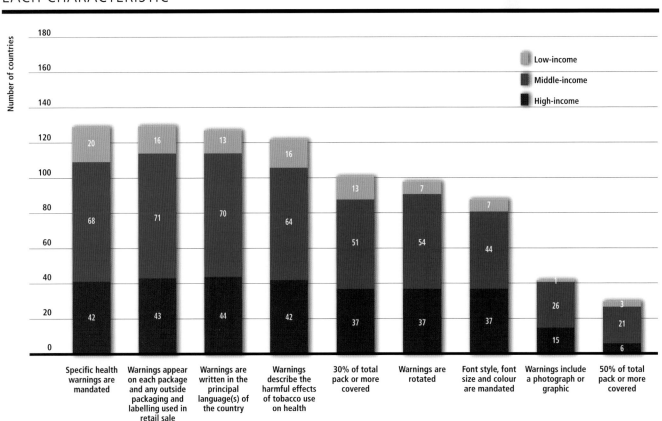

cigarettes, and 74 countries prohibit them on smokeless tobacco products.

Smokeless tobacco products are less likely to have health warning labels

In countries where there is widespread use of smokeless tobacco products, warning labels affixed directly to these products would provide tobacco users with important health information.

Smokeless tobacco products are included in the health warning legislation of 126 countries, either explicitly or by referring to all tobacco products inclusively.

As is the case with manufactured cigarettes, many of these countries do not require warning labels that incorporate best-practice characteristics for smokeless tobacco products. Only seven countries have adopted the strongest level of regulations for smokeless tobacco warnings, including warning labels that cover at least 50% of the packaging: Chile, Egypt, Iran, Mexico, Panama, Peru and Uruguay.

The two most common features of smokeless tobacco legislation among these 126 countries are that warnings should appear on each pack as well as on outside packaging and be in the countries' principal language(s). The least commonly reported feature is

that warnings include a photograph or pictorial graphic.

In the South-East Asia Region (SEAR), where smokeless tobacco products are extensively used, seven of 11 countries reported smokeless tobacco use for this report. However, only six SEAR countries (Bhutan, Democratic People's Republic of Korea, India, Maldives, Nepal and Sri Lanka) have legislation requiring health warnings on smokeless tobacco packaging. None of the SEAR countries currently meets the best-practice level for health warnings on smokeless tobacco products.

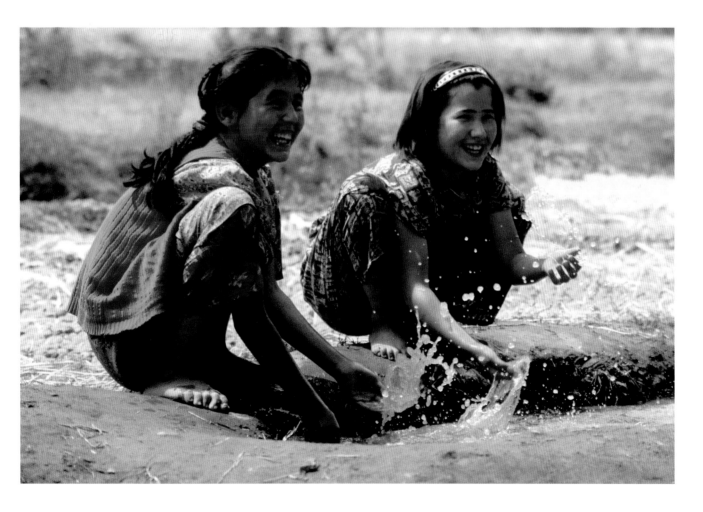

Anti-tobacco mass media campaigns

Nearly 28% of the world's population is exposed to effective anti-tobacco mass media campaigns

Anti-tobacco mass media campaigns were assessed for the first time for this report. There are currently 23 countries, with a total of more than 1.9 billion people representing 28% of the world's population, that have conducted media campaigns that were national in scope and that incorporated all appropriate characteristics:

- The campaign was part of a comprehensive government tobacco control programme.
- The campaign utilized media planning strategies.
- Research was conducted to develop campaign messaging and materials.

- Campaign materials were pre-tested before use.
- The campaign was monitored during implementation to ensure that materials were used as planned.
- The campaign was evaluated to assess impact.
- Earned media was used as an adjunct to the campaign.

Another 30 countries have conducted campaigns that incorporate at least five of the seven listed characteristics.

High-income countries, which are expected to have the necessary financial resources to run media campaigns, are the most likely to have carried out campaigns featuring most of these characteristics, although many

middle- and low-income countries have also run effective campaigns that incorporate most or all of the listed characteristics. However, over half of all countries reporting data did not run any national-level media campaigns during the survey period (January 2009 through August 2010).

More than a third of all countries have conducted a national anti-tobacco mass media campaign with at least some key characteristics

Of the seven campaign characteristics assessed for report categories, the most commonly implemented component was that the campaign utilized media planning

CHARACTERISTICS OF MASS MEDIA CAMPAIGNS, BY INCOME GROUP OF COUNTRY

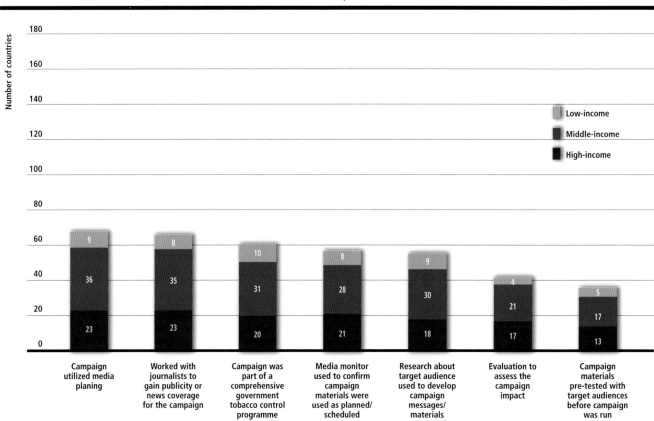

MASS MEDIA CAMPAIGNS

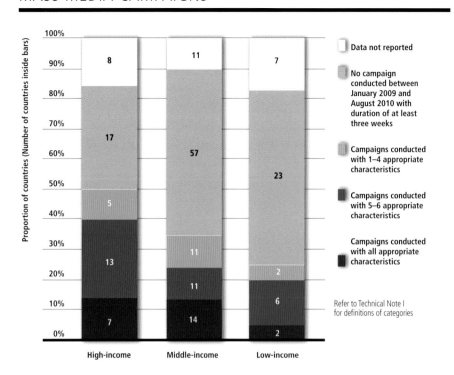

Proportion of countries (Number of countries inside bars)

High-income — 8, 17, 5, 13, 7
Middle-income — 11, 57, 11, 11, 14
Low-income — 7, 23, 2, 6, 2

Legend:
- Data not reported
- No campaign conducted between January 2009 and August 2010 with duration of at least three weeks
- Campaigns conducted with 1–4 appropriate characteristics
- Campaigns conducted with 5–6 appropriate characteristics
- Campaigns conducted with all appropriate characteristics

Refer to Technical Note I for definitions of categories

Over 60 countries reported that their campaigns were conducted as part of a comprehensive national tobacco control programme, a strategy that maximizes campaign effectiveness.

ANTI-TOBACCO MASS MEDIA CAMPAIGNS – HIGHEST ACHIEVING COUNTRIES, 2010

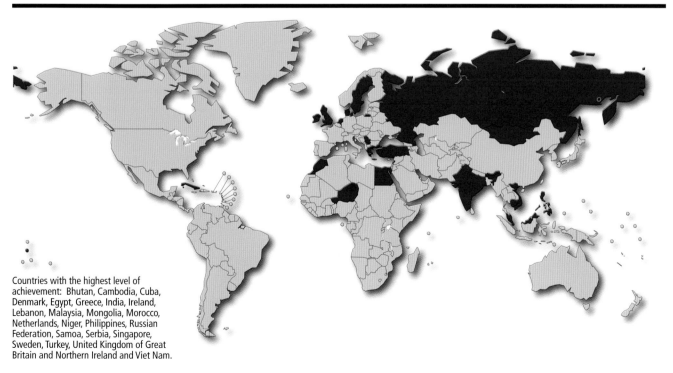

Countries with the highest level of achievement: Bhutan, Cambodia, Cuba, Denmark, Egypt, Greece, India, Ireland, Lebanon, Malaysia, Mongolia, Morocco, Netherlands, Niger, Philippines, Russian Federation, Samoa, Serbia, Singapore, Sweden, Turkey, United Kingdom of Great Britain and Northern Ireland and Viet Nam.

strategies. Media planning is an important campaign element, as it helps to ensure that the public is exposed to the campaign at times and in places where it will have the greatest impact.

Encouragingly, over 60 countries reported that their campaigns were run as part of a comprehensive national tobacco control programme, a strategy that maximizes campaign effectiveness. This element was the most frequently named campaign characteristic among low-income countries, with all 10 of those implementing a campaign doing so as part of a comprehensive national tobacco control programme.

The least frequently mentioned characteristics were evaluation to assess campaign impact and pre-testing of materials prior to conducting campaigns.

Warning about the harms of smoking and second-hand smoke exposure are frequent campaign objectives

In 48 countries, the primary campaign objective was to warn about the harms of smoking, making this the most commonly stated objective. Warning about the harms of second-hand smoke exposure was also a common campaign objective,

reported by 35 countries. Over two thirds of low-income countries reported warning about the dangers of tobacco use and warning about the harms of second-hand smoke exposure as their main campaign objectives. This is important because research shows that the health harms of smoking and second-hand smoke exposure are often not well understood in low-income countries, and thus more education is needed.

Stopping youth from using tobacco was also a common campaign objective, reported by 35 countries. Because general campaign messaging is also effective at reaching youth, specific targeting of youth may not

Television advertising is the most commonly employed type of media for anti-tobacco mass media campaigns.

MEDIA USED FOR ANTI-TOBACCO MASS MEDIA CAMPAIGNS

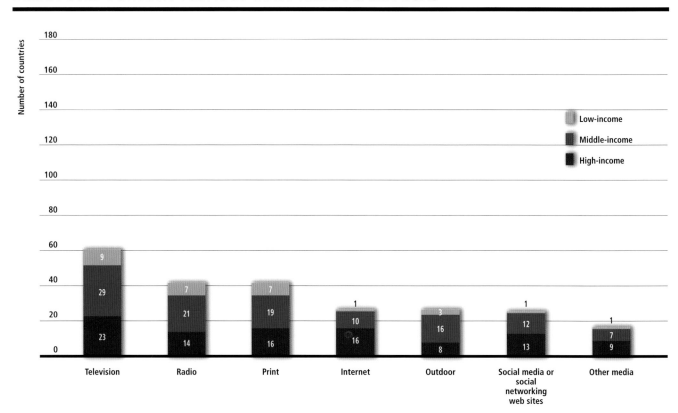

be necessary if strong campaigns that reach the entire country are in place.

Broadcast media are the most commonly used for campaigns

Television advertising is the most commonly employed type of media in which to run anti-tobacco advertising campaigns, used by 61 countries, and radio is also widely used (42 countries). Because broadcast media tend to have the widest audience reach, their use facilitates greater exposure of anti-tobacco messaging to the public.

Print media are also widely used, with 42 counties using print advertising as part of their campaigns. Other media types, which have lower population reach, tend to be used less frequently; some of these (e.g. Internet or social media) require further exploration. The number of countries using these newer media technologies for anti-tobacco campaigns can be expected to increase in the future as their use becomes more widespread.

Twenty-three countries, totalling more than 1.9 billion people, have conducted national anti-tobacco mass media campaigns.

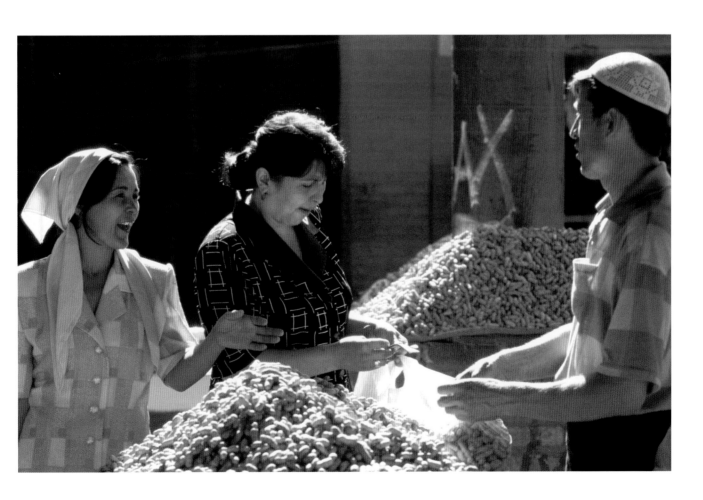

Uruguay mandates pictorial warning labels that cover most of the package, in line with WHO FCTC requirements

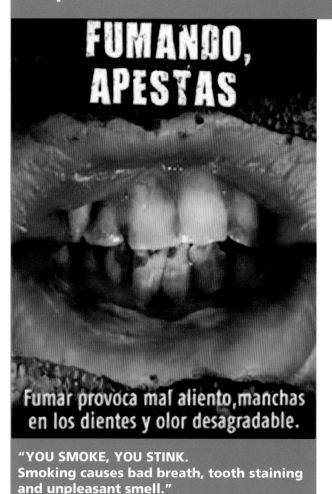

FUMANDO, APESTAS

Fumar provoca mal aliento, manchas en los dientes y olor desagradable.

**"YOU SMOKE, YOU STINK.
Smoking causes bad breath, tooth staining and unpleasant smell."**

Uruguay has required health warning labels on cigarette packages for nearly 30 years. However, the first labels were considered weak and ineffective because they were small, text-only warnings that were not displayed prominently on the packaging and included only a nonspecific message: "Smoking is harmful to health". By 2000, however, Uruguay's Health Ministry began to coordinate efforts to implement more effective tobacco control measures.

As a result, in 2003 health warnings were modified to feature more direct and specific messaging that read: "Smoking may cause cancer, lung and heart disease" and "Smoking when pregnant harms your baby". Although improved, the warnings continued to be small, not prominently displayed, and used no pictures. By 2005, after ratifying the WHO FCTC, Uruguay increased the size of the warning labels to cover half of the main display areas on both the front and back of the packaging, but still included no pictures.

In March 2005 a major boost was given to tobacco control policy in the country, and the Health Ministry established a formal national tobacco control programme. Within months, pictures were added to health warning labels, and misleading terms such as "light", "ultra light" or "mild" were prohibited. In 2008, the policy was further strengthened according to WHO FCTC Article 11 to allow only one presentation per brand in order to ensure that tobacco product packaging and labelling do not promote a tobacco product by any means that are false or misleading, including designs, colours, or any other signs that may create the false impression that one tobacco product is less harmful than another. In 2009, the size of warning labels was increased to 80% of primary pack surface areas. Results from the Global Adult Tobacco Survey show that nearly half of Uruguay's smokers are considering quitting because of these enhanced health warnings.

In view of the effectiveness of labelling provisions, a tobacco company has challenged the laws in a particularly alarming and aggressive fashion by initiating international arbitration to overturn them. In early 2010, an international tobacco company announced that it had filed for arbitration at the World Bank's International Centre for Settlement of Investment Disputes, claiming that Uruguay has violated its bilateral investment agreement with Switzerland. The Government of Uruguay, with support from international tobacco control advocates, is actively defending the laws.

Countries with already strong health warning label requirements can strengthen them even further. Canada, which was the first country to require graphic pictorial labels and which currently mandates that they cover 50% of the front and back of packs, has proposed increasing label size to 75% of primary pack surface areas. Label content would also be augmented with 16 new graphic health warnings that would rotate, eight new health information messages with new colour and graphic elements, and promotion of a new nationwide toll-free quit line number and web portal. Another example of a country that wants to further increase the impact of its pictorial health warnings is Australia: The Parliament is expected to adopt a bill to require generic tobacco packaging in 2011, which would make Australia the first country to mandate generic packaging beginning in July 2012.

Djibouti implements strong pictorial health warning labels to meet public demand for information

Due to growing demand for information about the health harms of tobacco, the tobacco control unit within Djibouti's Ministry of Health faced many challenges, including the high costs of producing informational materials and launching large-scale education and communication efforts. To bring health information directly to the public at the lowest possible cost and align with WHO FCTC requirements, the country chose to implement strong health warning labels on tobacco packaging.

With the support of international tobacco control experts and in-country organizations, a variety of warning label images was pre-tested. Ultimately, 11 different labels were selected that feature powerful images intended to raise awareness among smokers of both the health hazards to themselves and the risks of second-hand tobacco smoke exposure to others. Additionally, despite tobacco industry objections, Djibouti mandated pictorial labels covering 50% of both the front and back of packages, as well as health messages on the package sides.

The health warnings were implemented in 2009, at no cost to the country's government. Monitoring the impact of these new labels demonstrated that the labels were effective: within the first year, sales of tobacco products incorporating "strong" images on pack warning labels were substantially lower than sales of products containing "softer" images. As a result, Djibouti has proposed a new series of even stronger warning label images to begin in 2012. There is no requirement for health warning labels on tobacco products used for water pipe smoking; an increase in water pipe use indicates a need to expand warning labels to these products.

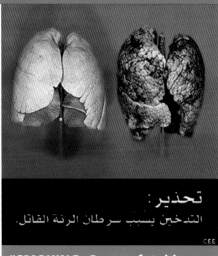

"SMOKING: Causes fatal lung cancer."

Mauritius implements large pictorial pack warning labels

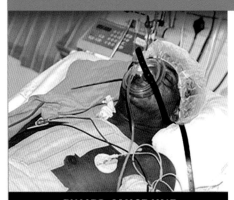

FUMER CAUSE UNE MORT LENTE ET DOULOUREUSE

"Smoking causes a long and painful death"

Tobacco use is a leading factor in the increasing epidemic of noncommunicable diseases in Mauritius. As part of a comprehensive five-year tobacco control plan, the country adopted new tobacco regulations in November 2008, becoming the first and so far only country in Africa to mandate pictorial health warnings on cigarette packs. These warnings are among the largest and most prominent in the world, occupying on average 65% of the total principal surface areas of the pack.

A set of eight rotating pictorial health warnings, which feature themes of addictiveness, second-hand smoke and health hazards, were selected based on survey findings and best-practice experiences of other countries. The warnings were pre-tested using qualitative techniques to assess their appropriateness, clarity, acceptance, pertinence and appeal, as well as respect for the needs of the country's multicultural and multiethnic society.

Evaluation showed that the new pictorial warning labels were substantially more effective than the previous text-only warnings. Many more smokers reported that they noticed the new warning labels and looked at them more often, that the warning labels made them more likely to feel uncomfortable or alarmed, and that they increased their likelihood of reducing consumption or wanting to quit altogether. Mauritius intends to introduce a new set of pictorial health warnings in the future to sustain continued attention and interest, and will work to ensure that they are consistent with its comprehensive package of tobacco prevention and control strategies.

Turkey increases free radio and television time for anti-tobacco advertising

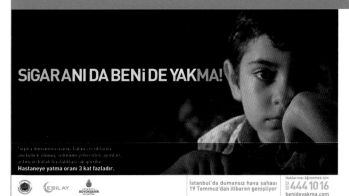

SİGARANI DA BENİ DE YAKMA!

"When you light up you ruin me!"

In 2003, the head of the Turkish parliamentarian health commission began drafting new tobacco control legislation. A provision was included to mandate broadcasts of anti-tobacco educational programming during daytime and early evening hours (8:00–22:00) so that messaging would reach increased numbers of adults and also be more likely to reach children. A further provision of the law requires that a minimum of 30 minutes per month be aired during evening prime time hours (17:00–22:00), which are the most heavily viewed programming slots.

Since 1996, Turkey has mandated that radio and television stations provide a minimum of 90 minutes of free air time every month for anti-tobacco educational programming and advertising. However, television channels generally showed these advertisements very early in the morning or late at night, and thus few people were exposed to their anti-tobacco messages.

Although there have been some enforcement problems due to the large number of television and radio channels in Turkey, the free air time is now being used for pre-tested effective anti-tobacco advertising. Other countries are currently examining the Turkish tobacco control legislation using the mandatory free air time requirements as a model for drafting national tobacco control legislation.

Key regions of the Russian Federation implement hard-hitting anti-tobacco advertising as a catalyst for change

With 43 million tobacco users, the Russian Federation has among the highest rates of smoking in the world – 60% of men and 20% of women. Although the Ministry of Health did not have a mandate for overarching tobacco control until late 2010, tobacco control experts started to lay the groundwork for hard-hitting anti-tobacco advertising campaigns beginning in 2008.

As part of a strategy to encourage the government to implement a national tobacco control programme, key regions in the Russian Federation were evaluated based on population size, available resources and political will necessary to conduct media campaigns. Advertising materials shown to be effective in other countries were adapted, and technical assistance was provided to regional governments in Chuvashia, Krasnodarsk, Moscow and Samara, among others, which aired the advertising campaigns.

Government involvement assured a wide reach for the campaign messaging via deeply discounted media buys as well as through earned media provided at no cost. For example, in Moscow, a US$ 175 000 advertising purchase resulted in media exposure worth nearly US$ 2.5 million. Evaluations in Moscow showed that the campaign increased the likelihood that people would talk about smoking and its harms and that smokers would consider quitting. The success of these campaigns also prompted several municipal and regional governments to push for smoke-free initiatives and laws, and in September 2010 the Russian Federation adopted a comprehensive national tobacco control strategy.

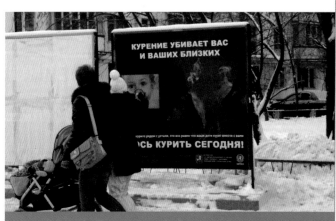

"Smoking kills you and those who are dear to you — Quit smoking today!"

Indian government airs campaign to highlight dangers of smokeless tobacco

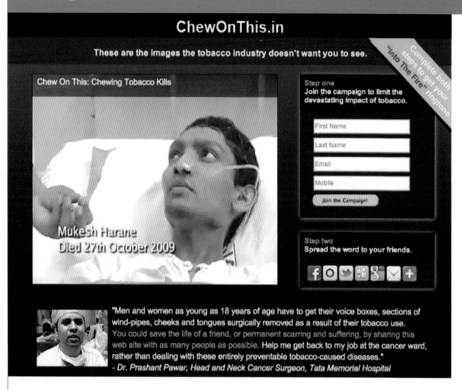

included hard-hitting footage of patients with tobacco-related cancers and featured an oral cancer surgeon describing the disfigurements suffered by tobacco chewers. The campaign was also adapted for northeastern Indian audiences and ran for eight weeks in early 2010. An evaluation of the campaign showed high recall and impact (75).

The second phase of the campaign against smokeless tobacco aired on television and radio from January to March 2011 in 16 languages. It featured Mukesh Harane, a 24-year-old smokeless tobacco user who died from oral cancer caused by chewing tobacco, and showed other patients at Tata Memorial Hospital in Mumbai who suffered from disfiguring and deadly cancers attributable to its use. The campaign generated considerable press coverage and helped bring facts about the smokeless tobacco epidemic in the country to the forefront.

Within its National Tobacco Control Programme, the Government of India allocates approximately US$ 5 million annually to anti-tobacco mass media campaigns. Based on increasing evidence, including the recent Global Adult Tobacco Survey that shows smokeless tobacco is used by more than a quarter of all adults in India, one of the most recent campaigns highlights the harmful effects of smokeless tobacco use.

The campaign was run in three 6-week phases for more than a year to warn the public about the dangers of smokeless tobacco use. The first phase of the campaign, which aired on television and radio in November and December 2009 in 11 local languages,

A web site (http://www.chewonthis.in) has been developed and launched jointly by the Ministry of Health and Family Welfare and Tata Memorial Hospital as an advocacy platform to highlight the dangers of smokeless tobacco products. An innovative mobile technology using text messaging has also been used to supplement television and radio advertising on the harms of smokeless tobacco use.

Enforce bans on tobacco advertising, promotion and sponsorship

The WHO Framework Convention on Tobacco Control states (1): Article 13: … a comprehensive ban on advertising, promotion and sponsorship would reduce the consumption of tobacco products. Each Party shall … undertake a comprehensive ban of all tobacco advertising, promotion and sponsorship.

start (143). Tobacco advertising, promotion and sponsorship normalize tobacco use and impede efforts to educate people about its harms (143). Complete bans on these activities block the industry's ability to continue marketing to young people who have not yet started to use tobacco, and to adult tobacco users who want to quit (143).

consumption by about 7%, independent of other tobacco control interventions (143), with some countries experiencing a decline in consumption of up to 16% (143).

Bans need to be complete and well enforced

Bans must be comprehensive: partial bans have little or no effect (143), and usually do not include indirect forms of marketing (143). Voluntary restrictions are ineffective; well-drafted and well-enforced legislation is required because the tobacco industry will circumvent advertising bans (143).

Comprehensive bans are necessary

Marketing of tobacco products encourages current smokers to smoke more, decreases their motivation to quit, and urges youth to

Bans are effective

Both direct and indirect advertising should be banned (143). A comprehensive ban on all tobacco advertising, promotion and sponsorship could decrease tobacco

BANS ON ADVERTISING, PROMOTION AND SPONSORSHIP

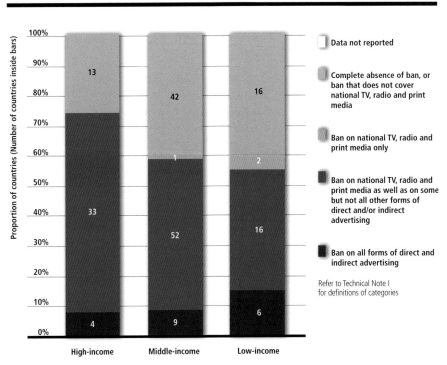

RECENT ACHIEVEMENTS AND DEVELOPMENTS

Increased media scrutiny of tobacco industry activities can highlight violations of advertising bans and noncompliance with the WHO FCTC as well as shape public opinion about event sponsorships. Unfavourable media coverage in China, together with advocacy by the Chinese health sector and tobacco control advocates, led to cancellation of tobacco sponsorships of several high-profile events, including the 2010 Shanghai World Expo (155). To avoid similar negative publicity, and to honour China's obligations under the WHO FCTC and to promote public health through sport, the 16th Asian Games held in November 2010 in Guangzhou were made

completely smoke-free from their inception, including a total ban on tobacco company sponsorships and the advertising and sale of tobacco products (156).

In Indonesia, tobacco control advocates enlisted the media as active partners. Outreach to journalists generated news coverage publicizing tobacco company event sponsorships, including high-profile concerts by popular singers such as Alicia Keys and Kelly Clarkson, and the resulting negative publicity forced the sponsorships to be withdrawn (157).

A comprehensive ban on all tobacco advertising, promotion and sponsorship could decrease tobacco consumption by about 7%, independent of other tobacco control interventions, with some countries experiencing a decline in consumption of up to 16%.

ENFORCE BANS ON TOBACCO ADVERTISING, PROMOTION AND SPONSORSHIP – HIGHEST ACHIEVING COUNTRIES, 2010

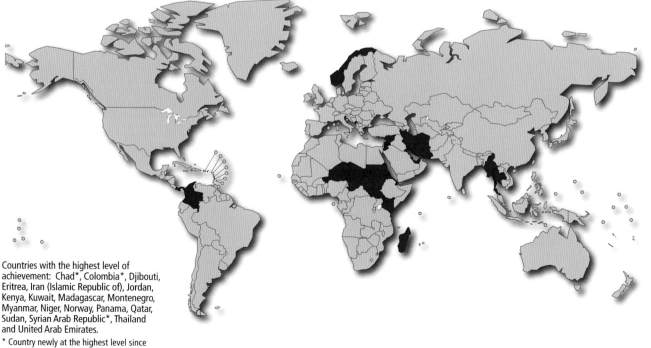

Countries with the highest level of achievement: Chad*, Colombia*, Djibouti, Eritrea, Iran (Islamic Republic of), Jordan, Kenya, Kuwait, Madagascar, Montenegro, Myanmar, Niger, Norway, Panama, Qatar, Sudan, Syrian Arab Republic*, Thailand and United Arab Emirates.

* Country newly at the highest level since 31 December 2008.

Progress is slow in comprehensively banning tobacco advertising, promotion and sponsorship

Between 2008 and 2010, three additional countries (Chad, Colombia and the Syrian Arab Republic) enacted comprehensive bans on tobacco advertising, promotion and sponsorship that covered all forms of direct as well as indirect advertising. There are now 19 countries with 425 million people, representing 6% of the world's population, who are now fully protected against tobacco industry marketing tactics, 80 million more than in 2008. Of these 19 countries, nine are classified as middle-income, six as low-income, and four as high-income.

An additional 101 countries ban national television, radio and print tobacco advertising, as well as some but not all other forms of direct and/or indirect advertising. However, this level of ban is still insufficient to protect people from tobacco advertising and marketing. Another 74 countries (38% of all countries) currently do not have any restrictions at all on tobacco advertising, promotion and sponsorship or have very minimal restrictions.

Bans must be comprehensive: partial bans have little or no effect, and usually do not include indirect forms of marketing.

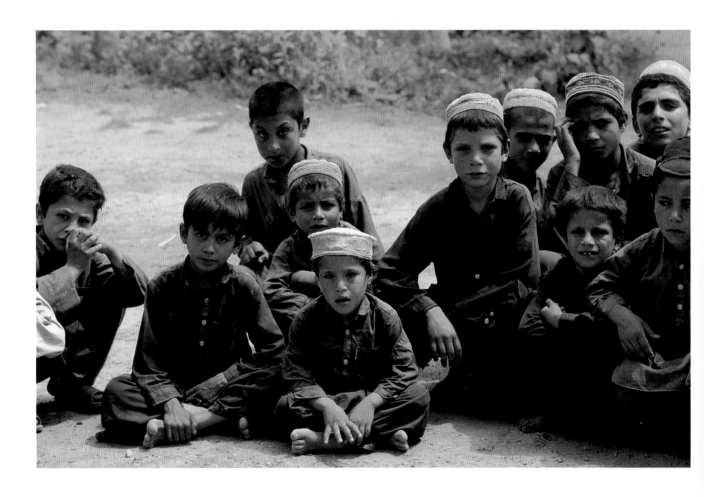

Chittagong City, Bangladesh, passes a strong subnational advertising ban

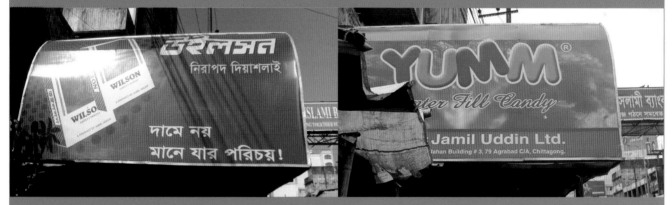

Before ban.

After ban.

Chittagong City, population 4 million, is Bangladesh's second largest city. It has an active network of tobacco control advocacy organizations that work closely with local government to advance the tobacco control agenda. In 2010, this advocacy work helped lead the Chittagong City government to enact a ban on all tobacco advertising, including advertising indirectly through surrogates and brand extensions such as lighters featuring cigarette brands.

Although there is an existing national ban on tobacco billboard advertising, the law does not explicitly cover indirect advertising, point-of-sale marketing, or other promotional activities, and overall enforcement is suboptimal. The Chittagong City regulations expand and strengthen the national law by banning all tobacco billboard advertising and creating a clear mechanism for enforcement.

All tobacco billboard advertising was removed immediately upon passage of the law, and other forms of advertising including at the point of sale were eliminated shortly thereafter. Tobacco control advocacy groups continue to work with local government agencies to ensure effective enforcement of the ban.

There are 425 million people in 19 countries, representing 6% of the world's population, who are now fully protected against tobacco industry marketing tactics, 80 million more than in 2008. Of these 19 countries, nearly all are low- or middle-income.

mpower Raise taxes on tobacco

The WHO Framework Convention on Tobacco Control states (1): Article 6: … price and tax measures are an effective and important means of reducing tobacco consumption … [Parties] … should … adopt … measures which may include: … tax policies and … price policies on tobacco products so as to contribute to the health objectives aimed at reducing tobacco consumption. Article 15: …elimination of all forms of illicit trade in tobacco products, including smuggling, illicit manufacturing and counterfeiting … are essential components of tobacco control.

Increasing taxes is the best way to reduce tobacco use

Increasing tobacco prices through higher taxes is the most effective intervention to reduce tobacco use and encourage smokers to quit (143). Higher taxes are particularly effective in keeping youth from starting to smoke and reducing use among the poor (143). Each 10% increase in retail price reduces consumption by about 4% in high-income countries and up to 8% in low- and middle-income countries, with smoking prevalence reduced by about half those rates (14).

Higher taxes increase government revenues

Tobacco taxes are generally well accepted, and even supported by many smokers, because most people understand that tobacco use is harmful (143). Tax increases raise government revenues, which can be used for tobacco control and other important health and social programmes; allocating tax revenues in this way further increases popular support for raising taxes (143).

Strong tax administration improves compliance

Increased smuggling does not automatically follow tax increases; good governance is a more important determinant of smuggling than differences in tax rates (143). Countries should strengthen tax administration and customs enforcement capacity, particularly where there are high levels of smuggling and/or tax evasion (14).

Taxes must keep pace with inflation and incomes

Taxes should be increased periodically to offset the combined effects of inflation and increased incomes and purchasing power (143). If real cigarette prices do not rise faster than consumer purchasing power, tobacco becomes relatively more affordable and consumption increases (14).

TOTAL TAX ON CIGARETTES

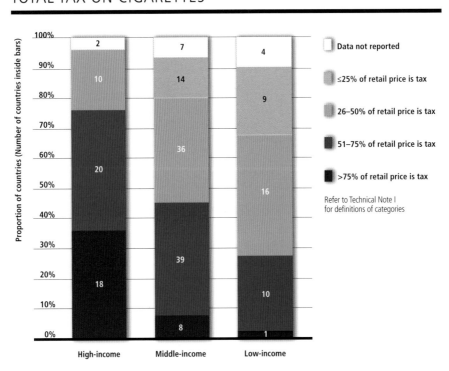

RECENT ACHIEVEMENTS AND DEVELOPMENTS

To assist countries to increase tobacco taxes and prices, WHO developed, in consultation with external experts, a *Technical Manual on Tobacco Tax Administration* (*158*) for use by all countries, and is conducting training workshops on tobacco taxation for finance ministry officials and technical experts in public finance in different regions.

The fourth session of the COP to the WHO FCTC established a working group to develop guidelines for the implementation of Article 6 (Price and tax measures to reduce the demand for tobacco) of the WHO FCTC (*159*). The COP also mandated the Intergovernmental Negotiating Body to continue negotiating a draft protocol to eliminate illicit trade in tobacco products, which the COP will consider for approval in 2012 (*159*).

Increasing tobacco prices through higher taxes is the most effective intervention to reduce tobacco use and encourage smokers to quit.

RAISE TAXES ON TOBACCO – HIGHEST ACHIEVING COUNTRIES AND TERRITORIES, 2010

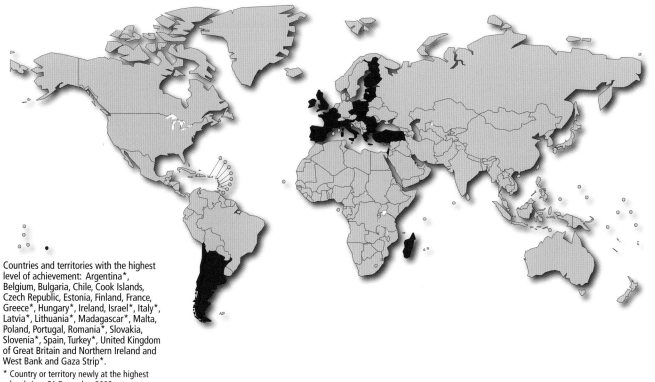

Countries and territories with the highest level of achievement: Argentina*, Belgium, Bulgaria, Chile, Cook Islands, Czech Republic, Estonia, Finland, France, Greece*, Hungary*, Ireland, Israel*, Italy*, Latvia*, Lithuania*, Madagascar*, Malta, Poland, Portugal, Romania*, Slovakia, Slovenia*, Spain, Turkey*, United Kingdom of Great Britain and Northern Ireland and West Bank and Gaza Strip*.

* Country or territory newly at the highest level since 31 December 2008.

Taxes in some countries are not keeping pace with increases in tobacco prices

There are now 26 countries and one territory that have total taxes constituting more than 75% of the retail price. Since 2008, there have been 11 countries and one territory (Argentina, Greece, Hungary, Israel, Italy, Latvia, Lithuania, Madagascar, Romania, Slovenia, Turkey and West Bank and Gaza Strip) that have increased tobacco taxes so that they constitute more than 75% of the retail price. However, six

countries that had tobacco taxation at that level in 2008 have by 2010 seen their share of taxes as a proportion of retail price fall below the 75% benchmark. This was not always caused by reductions in tax rates, but because taxes (primarily specific taxes set at a fixed amount) did not increase as prices increased. In addition, two countries formerly reported to levy taxes at this level (Cuba and Fiji) did not report data on taxes for 2010. As a result, there is a net increase of four countries/territories that now levy taxes at the recommended 75% level, with an increase of 115 million people newly

protected by tax legislation at the highest level since 2008, bringing the total to more than 539 million people representing 8% of the world's population.

High-income countries are more likely to levy taxes at sufficiently high levels so that they make up more than 75% of retail price; the same holds when the threshold level is reduced to 50%. However, only one low-income country currently levies taxes at 75% of the retail price, and less than 10% of middle-income countries do so.

Since 2008, there have been 11 countries and one territory that have increased tobacco taxes so that they constitute more than 75% of the retail price.

AVERAGE RETAIL PRICE AND TAXATION (EXCISE AND TOTAL) OF MOST SOLD BRANDS OF CIGARETTES, 2010

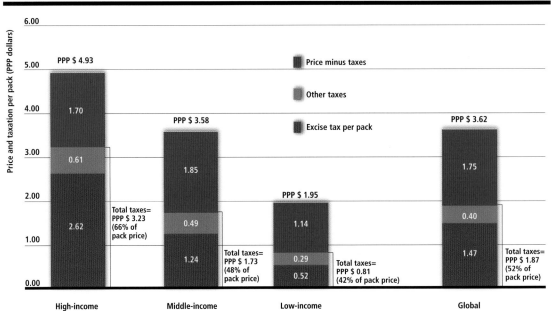

Note: Prices are expressed in Purchasing Power Parity (PPP) adjusted dollars or international dollars to account for differences in purchasing power across countries. Based on 45 high-income, 89 middle-income and 33 low-income countries with data on price of most sold brand, excise and other taxes and PPP conversion factors.

Egypt restructures and increases tobacco excise taxes and earmarks additional revenues to fund health programmes

In July 2010, Egypt's Ministry of Finance restructured its tax system for tobacco products to reduce tax avoidance, generate more tax revenues and improve public health by reducing tobacco consumption. The government eliminated its tiered tax system, replacing eight different rates based on price with a uniformly applied 40% ad valorem excise tax as well as a single specific tax rate of Egyptian £ 1.25 (approximately US$ 0.20) per pack of cigarettes. Taxes on loose tobacco were also increased by 100%.

Under the new system, total taxes per pack of cigarettes increased by an average of 87%, which increased the average retail price by an estimated 44%. This tax-induced price increase on cigarettes is expected to reduce cigarette consumption by 21% and smoking prevalence by more than 10%, and hence reduce the number of adult smokers by about 893 000 and prevent about 208 000 premature deaths.

The decision to increase tobacco taxes in Egypt was driven in part by government efforts to secure additional funds to overhaul health care and expand health insurance coverage (*160*). Egypt's approach to reaching the dual goals of reduced tobacco consumption and increased resources to spend on health can provide valuable lessons for other countries.

INCREASED TOBACCO TAXES WITH SIMPLIFIED STRUCTURE PREDICTED TO MORE THAN DOUBLE TAX REVENUES, REDUCE CONSUMPTION BY ONE FIFTH, AND REDUCE PREVALENCE BY OVER 10%

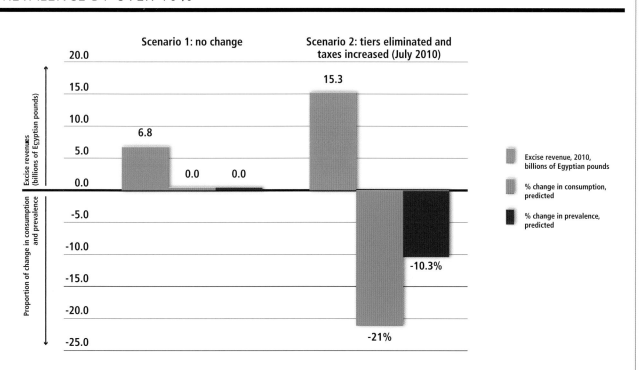

Note: The graph describes the predicted impact of two scenarios on excise revenues and tobacco use: 1) under Egypt's pre-2010 tiered system, and 2) the policy implemented in July 2010 – a change in tax structure (eliminating tiers) and a higher excise tax rate. Scenario 2 more than doubles excise revenues; it also results in higher prices and substantial reductions in cigarette consumption and the number of smokers.

National action is critical to achieve the vision of a tobacco-free world

The WHO Framework Convention on Tobacco Control states (1): Article 5: Each Party shall develop, implement, periodically update and review comprehensive multisectoral national tobacco control strategies, plans and programmes ... [and] establish or reinforce and finance a national coordinating mechanism or focal points for tobacco control. In addition, WHO FCTC Article 26.2 indicates that each Party shall provide financial support in respect of its national activities intended to achieve the objective of the Convention (1).

National programmes are needed to lead tobacco control efforts

Building national capacity to carry out an effective and sustainable national tobacco control programme (NTCP) is critical to reversing the tobacco epidemic (143). Strategic planning and leadership for the NTCP should occur centrally within the ministry of health (143). A national coordinating mechanism at a high level of government should be convened with an official mandate to develop tobacco control infrastructure and coordinate policy implementation (14).

In larger countries, the NTCP should be designed for flexible implementation by decentralizing authority to subnational levels so that interventions can more effectively reach the entire country (14). Since most tobacco control interventions are carried out at the local level, success depends on adequate resources and capacity building for local public health professionals and government leaders (14).

Tobacco use prevalence often differs across income, age, ethnic groups and by gender, indicating social inequity. As national tobacco control programmes are designed to reduce tobacco use, efforts to ensure that population subgroups with disproportionately high rates of tobacco use are reached by policies and programmes are essential (161).

Funding for tobacco control is inadequate

Each country's government must provide its NTCP with a steady source of funding at national and, where appropriate, subnational levels (143). Governments collect nearly US$ 133 billion in tobacco excise tax revenues each year, but spend less than US$ 1 billion combined on

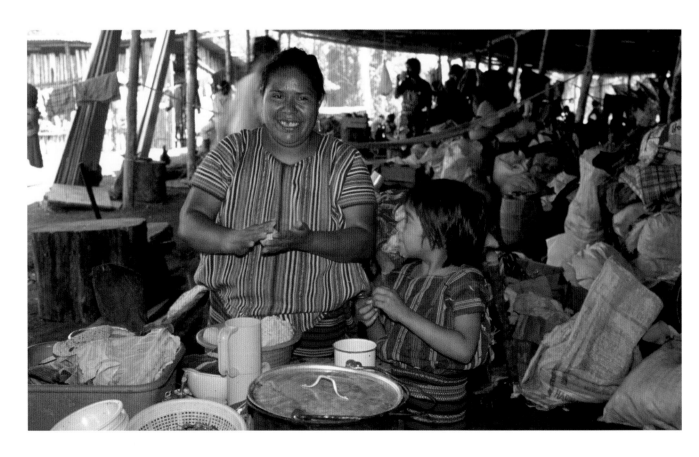

RECENT ACHIEVEMENTS AND DEVELOPMENTS

Within the past year, the Russian Federation has adopted its Concept for State Policy on Actions Against Tobacco Use for 2010–2015 in accordance with Article 5 of the WHO FCTC. A formal tobacco control programme mechanism has been established within the Ministry of Health and Social Development with responsibility for implementing a comprehensive national strategy that addresses all WHO FCTC requirements, including provisions on tax increases, advertising bans, smoke-free places, warning labels, cessation services, and public education activities that will include anti-tobacco mass media advertising. Specific programme goals have been set for 2015, including reducing tobacco use prevalence by 10–15% and reducing the number of people exposed to second-hand tobacco smoke by half (162).

Governments collect nearly US$ 133 billion in tobacco excise tax revenues each year, but spend less than US$ 1 billion combined on tobacco control – 97% of this amount are spent by high-income countries.

TOBACCO CONTROL IS UNDERFUNDED

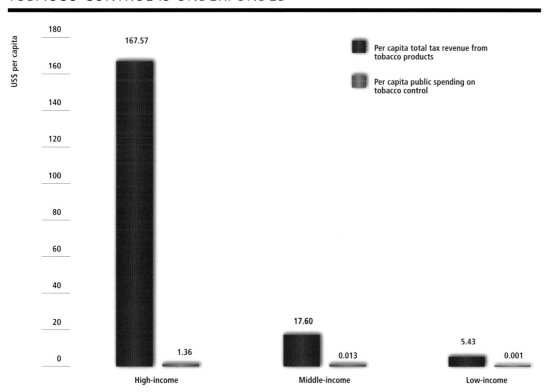

Note: Based on 51 countries with available tobacco excise revenue data for 2009; expenditure on tobacco control for several of these countries was estimated from figures reported between 2007 and 2010, adjusting for inflation. Tax revenues are tobacco product (or cigarette) excise revenues in 2009 for included countries. In a departure from the WHO Report on the Global Tobacco Epidemic, 2009, revenues here pertain to excises rather than all taxes on tobacco products. Due to this more stringent criterion, fewer countries are represented than in the 2009 report.

tobacco control– 97% of this amount are spent by high-income countries. While per capita excise revenues are about 124 times higher than tobacco control expenditures in high-income countries (US$ 167.57 per capita excise revenues vs US$ 1.36 per capita tobacco control expenditures), the difference is much higher in middle-income countries (excise revenues 1339 times higher than tobacco control expenditures) and low-income countries (excise revenues 4304 times higher than tobacco control expenditures).

This lack of funding is cause for extreme concern, as most countries have sufficient financial resources available to expand and strengthen NTCPs (143). Further tobacco tax increases can provide additional funding (143).

Tobacco control programmes need sufficient staffing

A NTCP with full-time, dedicated staff at both central and (where appropriate) subnational levels can provide highly effective leadership and administration of all programme initiatives (143). Successful tobacco control policy implementation also requires support from senior levels throughout government as well as technical experts and persons with expertise in planning and implementation (14). Most countries have developed tobacco control programmes or strategies, although staffing levels continue to be low.

Civil society must be involved with tobacco control efforts

NTCPs require logistic support and effective partnerships both within government and with all segments of civil society (143). Many nongovernmental organizations and other civil society groups have made great contributions to national and global tobacco control efforts; their continued involvement is essential to continued progress (143).

NATIONAL TOBACCO CONTROL PROGRAMMES

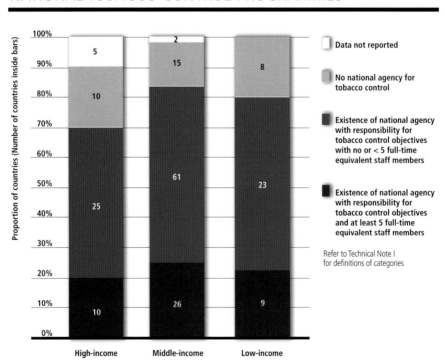

Most countries have a national tobacco control programme, but many do not staff them adequately

At least 154 countries have a national agency with some responsibility for tobacco control objectives, a slight increase over the results shown in the *WHO Report on the Global Tobacco Epidemic, 2009*, with low-and middle-income countries somewhat more likely to have such an agency than high-income countries. However, many countries do not sufficiently staff these agencies at a level that adequately supports tobacco control policy implementation. Only 20% of high-income countries and 24% of middle- and low-income countries have an agency with at least five full-time equivalent staff members, showing virtually no change from the previous survey period; just three countries (Burundi, Pakistan and Turkey) increased programme staffing to this level in the past two years. More than 30 countries either do not have a national tobacco control agency or have not established national objectives for tobacco control, which are critical foundations for complying with WHO FCTC treaty obligations.

Building national capacity to carry out an effective and sustainable national tobacco control programme is critical to reversing the tobacco epidemic.

Venezuela establishes an Intergovernmental Commission for Tobacco Control

Even prior to ratifying the WHO FCTC, the Bolivarian Republic of Venezuela had begun implementing most of the treaty's tobacco control measures. To further satisfy treaty requirements, the country's Ministry of Health established an Intergovernmental Commission for Tobacco Control to coordinate tobacco control programmes across all arms of government. The Ministries of Education, Environment, Interior Relations and Justice, Exterior Relations, Defence, Work and Social Security, and Economy and Finances joined this Commission, as did other government agencies including the National Integrated Service of the Customs and Tax Administration, National Antidrug Office, Rafael Rangel National Institute of Hygiene and the Institute of Prevention, Health and Labour Security.

Creation of the Commission shows strong support for tobacco control across all government sectors in Venezuela. A practical framework outlines responsibilities for each involved entity, such as monitoring and enforcement, taxation and finance, cessation support, and education, and provides a coordination mechanism for all activities and programmes. The Commission also cooperates with regional and international organizations including WHO, the Pan-American Health Organization (PAHO), Oras-Conhu, Mercosur and others.

The Commission's efforts in advancing tobacco control policies have resulted in bans on tobacco advertising and promotion, strong health warning label requirements for cigarette packs, tobacco tax rates that are among the highest in South America, and mechanisms to prevent smuggling. Continued coordination of the work being done by the Commission's constituent organizations is intended to result in even stronger tobacco control measures in Venezuela in the future.

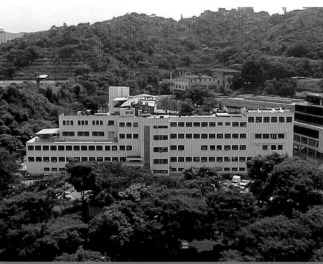

Ministry of Popular Power for Health and Social Protection

Conclusion

The WHO FCTC demonstrates continued global commitment to decisive action against the global tobacco epidemic, which kills millions of people and costs hundreds of billions of dollars each year. A total of 173 Parties to the WHO FCTC, covering about 87% of the world's population, have made a legally binding commitment to implement effective tobacco control policies. The WHO FCTC provides countries with the necessary tobacco control tools that, when implemented and enforced, will reduce tobacco use and save lives.

The status of the MPOWER measures presented in this *WHO Report on the Global Tobacco Epidemic, 2011* show that it is possible for any country, regardless of political structure or income level, to implement an effective tobacco control programme to reduce tobacco use.

- In total, nearly 3.8 billion people, or 55% of the world's population, are now covered by at least one of the measures at the highest level of achievement. More than one billion people (17% of the world's population) are covered by two or more measures at the highest level.

- More than 1.1 billion people have been newly protected by at least one tobacco control measure applied nationally at the highest level since 2008, with progress in all MPOWER measures. Mass media campaigns, an MPOWER measure assessed for the first time for this report, were conducted in 23 countries, comprising a significant 1.9 billion people, airing a best-practice anti-tobacco mass media campaign in 2009 or 2010.

- The greatest progress as measured by population coverage has been in the area of health warnings on tobacco packaging; three more countries with a total population of 458 million have enacted pack labelling laws at the highest level.

- Although subnational mass media campaigns were not formally assessed, it is likely that a substantial number of people were exposed to anti-tobacco advertising conducted at the local level.

- National-level smoke-free laws covering all public places and workplaces have been newly enacted by 16 countries with a total of 385 million people; an additional 100 million people are newly

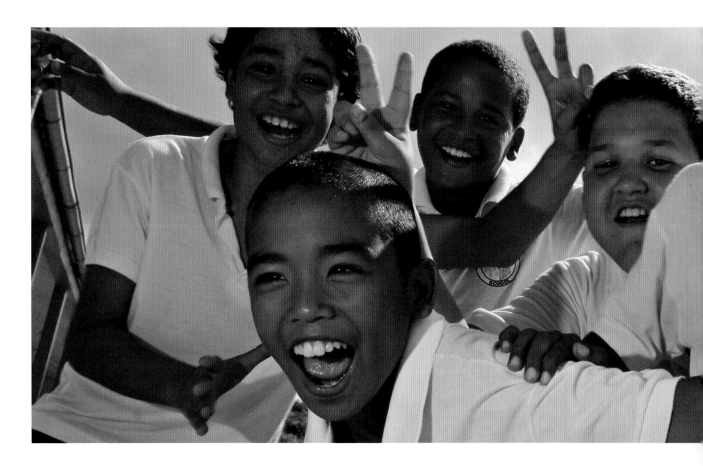

protected by comprehensive smoke-free laws at the subnational level.

- Comprehensive services to help people quit tobacco use have been applied by one additional country, with a total population of 76 million.
- Complete bans on all tobacco advertising, promotion and sponsorship are now in place in three more countries, with a total population of 80 million.
- An additional 115 million people are now living in countries with the recommended minimum tobacco taxes, and 26 countries and one territory now have taxes constituting the recommended minimum of 75% of retail price.
- Despite the progress being made by countries in levying revenue-generating tobacco taxes, governments still

inadequately fund tobacco control activities. Governments collect nearly US$ 133 billion in tobacco excise tax revenues, but spend less than US$ 1 billion on tobacco control, a deficit that is most evident in low- and middle-income countries.

The progress in reaching the highest level of the MPOWER measures is a sign of the growing success of the WHO FCTC and provides strong evidence that there is political will for tobacco control on both national and global levels, which can be harnessed to great effect. Many countries have made significant progress in fighting the epidemic of tobacco use, and can be looked to as models for action by those countries that have not as yet adopted these measures. Countries must continue to

expand and intensify their tobacco control efforts, ensuring they have both the financial means and political commitment to support effective and sustainable programmes.

Although there has been substantial progress on tobacco control in many countries, more work needs to be done. The successes already achieved can and must be expanded upon so that all people worldwide are fully protected against the harms of tobacco use.

Continued progress will stop millions of people from dying each year from preventable tobacco-related illness, and save hundreds of billions of dollars a year in avoidable health-care expenditures and productivity losses. It is up to us to make sure that this occurs.

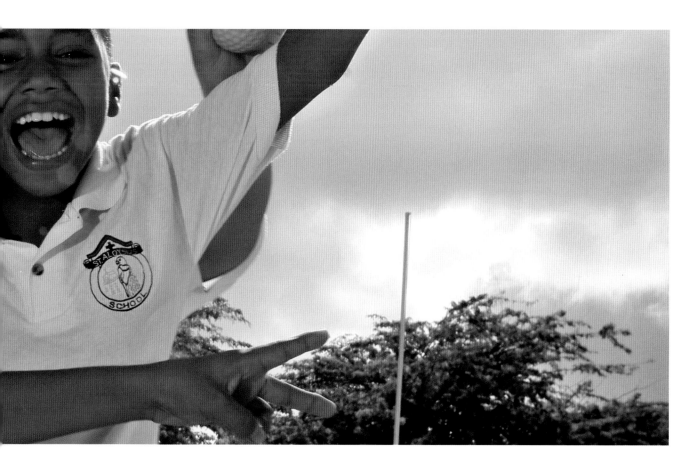

References

1. *WHO Framework Convention on Tobacco Control*. Geneva, World Health Organization, 2003 (updated 2004, 2005; http://www.who.int/tobacco/framework/WHO_FCTC_english.pdf, accessed 12 April 2011).

2. *Guidelines for implementation of Article 11 of the WHO Framework Convention on Tobacco Control (Packaging and labelling of tobacco products)*. Geneva, World Health Organization, 2008 (http://www.who.int/fctc/guidelines/article_11.pdf, accessed 12 April 2011).

3. *2008–2013 Action Plan for the Global Strategy for the Prevention and Control of Noncommunicable Diseases*. Geneva, World Health Organization, 2008 (http://www.who.int/nmh/Actionplan-PC-NCD-2008.pdf, accessed 12 April 2011).

4. *Guidelines for implementation of Article 12 of the WHO Framework Convention on Tobacco Control (Education, communication, training and public awareness)*. Geneva, World Health Organization, 2010 (http://www.who.int/fctc/guidelines/Decision.pdf, accessed 12 April 2011).

5. Chapman S et al. Ensuring smokers are adequately informed: reflections on consumer rights, manufacturer responsibilities, and policy implications. *Tobacco Control*, 2005, 14(Suppl. 2):ii8–ii13.

6. Hammond D et al. Effectiveness of cigarette warning labels in informing smokers about the risks of smoking: findings from the International Tobacco Control (ITC) Four Country Survey. *Tobacco Control*, 2006, 15(Suppl. 3):iii19–iii25.

7. *Reducing the health consequences of smoking: 25 years of progress. A report of the Surgeon General*. Rockville, MD, Center for Chronic Disease Prevention and Health Promotion, Office on Smoking and Health, 1989.

8. Siahpush M et al. Socioeconomic and country variations in knowledge of health risks of tobacco smoking and toxic constituents of smoke: results from the 2002 International Tobacco Control (ITC) Four Country Survey. *Tobacco Control*, 2006, 15(Suppl. 3):iii65–iii70.

9. *Tobacco: deadly in any form or disguise*. Geneva, World Health Organization, 2006 (http://www.who.int/tobacco/communications/events/wntd/2006/Tfi_Rapport.pdf, accessed 12 April 2011).

10. Borland R et al. What happened to smokers' beliefs about light cigarettes when "light/mild" brand descriptors were banned in the UK? Findings from the International Tobacco Control (ITC) Four Country Survey. *Tobacco Control*, 2008, 17:256–262.

11. Borland R et al. Use of and beliefs about light cigarettes in four countries. Findings from the International Tobacco Control Policy Evaluation Survey. *Nicotine & Tobacco Research*, 2004, 6(Suppl. 3):S311–S321.

12. *The health consequences of involuntary exposure to tobacco smoke: a report of the Surgeon General*. Atlanta, GA, US Department of Health and Human Services, Centers for Disease Control and Prevention, Coordinating Center for Health Promotion, National Center for Chronic Disease Prevention and Health Promotion, Office on Smoking and Health, 2006 (http://www.surgeongeneral.gov/library/secondhandsmoke/report/index.html, accessed 12 April 2011).

13. Romer D et al. The Catch-22 of Smoking and Quitting. In: Slovic P, ed. Smoking – *Risk, Perception, and Policy*. Thousand Oaks, CA, Sage, 2001.

14. *MPOWER: a policy package to reverse the tobacco epidemic*. Geneva, World Health Organization, 2008 (http://www.who.int/tobacco/mpower/mpower_english.pdf, accessed 12 April 2011).

15. *Youth and tobacco: preventing tobacco use among young people. A report of the Surgeon General*. Rockville, MD, US Department of Health and Human Services, Centers for Disease Control and Prevention, National Center for Chronic Disease Prevention and Health Promotion, Office on Smoking and Health, 1994.

16. *The role of the media in promoting and reducing tobacco use*. Bethesda, MD, US Department of Health and Human Services, National Institutes of Health, National Cancer Institute, 2008 (Tobacco Control Monograph No. 19; NIH Pub. No. 07-6242).

17. Wiehe SE et al. A systematic review of school-based smoking prevention trials with long-term follow-up. *Journal of Adolescent Health*, 2005, 36:162–169.

18. Thomas R, Perera R. School-based programmes for preventing smoking. *Cochrane Database of Systematic Reviews*, 2006 (3)CD 001293.

19. Warner KE. The need for, and value of, a multi-level approach to disease prevention: the case for tobacco control. In: Smedley BD, Syme SL, eds. *Promoting health: intervention strategies from social and behavioral research*. Washington, DC, National Academies Press, 2000.

20. Difranza J et al. Cigarette package design: opportunities for disease prevention. *Tobacco Induced Diseases*, 2003, 1:97–109.

21. Freeman B et al. The case for the plain packaging of tobacco products. *Addiction*, 2008, 103:580–590.

22. Wakefield MA et al. How does increasingly plainer cigarette packaging influence adult smokers' perceptions about brand image? An experimental study. *Tobacco Control*, 2008, 17:416–421.

23. Borland R, Hill D. Initial impact of the new Australian tobacco health warnings on knowledge and beliefs. *Tobacco Control*, 1997, 6:317–325.

24. Borland R. Tobacco health warnings and smoking-related cognitions and behaviours. *Addiction*, 1997, 92:1427–1435.

25. Fathelrahman AI et al. Smokers' responses toward cigarette pack warning labels in predicting quit intention, stage of change, and self-efficacy. *Nicotine & Tobacco Research*, 2009, 11:248–253.

26. *Opinião pública*. 76% sao a favor que embalagens de cigarros tragam imagens que ilustram males provocados pelo fumo; 67% dos fumantes que viram as imagens afirmam terem sentido vontade de parar de fumar [76% are in favour of pictures on cigarette packs that illustrate the problems caused by smoking, 67% of smokers saw the pictures and say they made them want to stop smoking]. São Paulo, Datafolha Instituto de Pesquisas, 2002.

27. Thrasher JF et al. Smokers' reactions to cigarette package warnings with graphic imagery and with only text: a comparison between Mexico and Canada. *Salud Pública de México*, 2007, 49(Suppl. 2):S233–S240.

28. Borland R et al. Impact of graphic and text warnings on cigarette packs: findings from four countries over five years. *Tobacco Control*, 2009, 18:358–364.

29. Hammond D et al. Impact of the graphic Canadian warning labels on adult smoking behaviour. *Tobacco Control*, 2003, 12:391–395.

30. Hammond D et al. Tobacco denormalization and industry beliefs among smokers from four countries. *American Journal of Preventive Medicine*, 2006, 31:225–232.

31. Callery WE et al. The appeal of smokeless tobacco products among young Canadian smokers: the impact of pictorial health warnings and relative risk messages. *Nicotine & Tobacco Research*, 2011 (Epub ahead of print, 28 February).

32. Hammond D et al. Text and graphic warnings on cigarette packages: findings from the International Tobacco Control Four Country Study. *American Journal of Preventive Medicine*, 2007, 32:202–209.

33. Nimbarte A et al. Comparison of current US and Canadian cigarette pack warnings. *International Quarterly of Community Health Education*, 2005, 24:3–27.

34. O'Hegarty M et al. Young adults' perceptions of cigarette warning labels in the United States and Canada. *Preventing Chronic Disease*, 2007, 4:A27.

35. O'Hegarty M et al. Reactions of young adult smokers to warning labels on cigarette packages. *American Journal of Preventive Medicine*, 2006, 30:467–473.

36. Peters E et al. The impact and acceptability of Canadian-style cigarette warning labels among US smokers and nonsmokers. *Nicotine & Tobacco Research*, 2007,9:473–481.

37. Fong G et al. Effects of the Canadian graphic warning labels among high school students: a quasi-experimental longitudinal survey. Presentation at: The 2002 National Conference on Tobacco or Health, San Francisco, 20 November 2002 (http://ncth.confex.com/ncth/2002/techprogram/paper_6056.htm, accessed 12 April 2011).

38. Borland R et al. How reactions to cigarette packet health warnings influence quitting: findings from the ITC Four-Country survey. *Addiction*, 2009, 104:669–675.

39. Sobani Z et al. Graphic tobacco health warnings: which genre to choose? *International Journal of Tuberculosis and Lung Disease*, 2010, 14:356–361.

40. Miller CL et al. Response of mass media, tobacco industry and smokers to the introduction of graphic cigarette pack warnings in Australia. *European Journal of Public Health*, 2009, 19:644–649.

41. Hammond D et al. The impact of cigarette warning labels and smoke-free bylaws on smoking cessation: evidence from former smokers. *Canadian Journal of Public Health*, 2004, 95:201–204.

42. Hammond D et al. Graphic Canadian cigarette warning labels and adverse outcomes: evidence from Canadian smokers. *American Journal of Public Health*, 2004, 94:1442–1445.

43. *Graphic health warnings on tobacco packaging inspire smokers to quit the habit.* Singapore, Health Promotion Board, 2004 (Press Release; http://hpb.gov.sg/hpb/default.asp?TEMPORARY_DOCUMENT=2982&TEMPORARY_TEMPLATE=2, accessed 12 April 2011).

44. *The International Tobacco Control Policy Evaluation Project: Thailand.* Waterloo, ON, The International Tobacco Control Policy Evaluation Project, 2010 (http://www.itcproject.org/projects/thailand/thexecsummaryadults07pdf, accessed 12 April 2011).

45. *Evaluation of new warnings on cigarette packages.* Toronto, Environics Research Group for the Canadian Cancer Society, 2003 (http://www.cancer.ca/~/media/CCS/Canada%20wide/Files%20List/English%20files%20heading/pdf%20not%20in%20publications%20section/Environics%20study%20on%20cigarette%20warning%20labels%20-%20complete.ashx, accessed 12 April 2011).

46. Wilson N et al. Long-term benefit of increasing the prominence of a quitline number on cigarette packaging: 3 years of Quitline call data. *New Zealand Medical Journal*, 2010, 123:109–111.

47. Vardavas CI et al. Adolescents' perceived effectiveness of the proposed European graphic tobacco warning labels. *European Journal of Public Health*, 2009, 19:212–217.

48. White V et al. Do graphic health warning labels have an impact on adolescents' smoking-related beliefs and behaviours? *Addiction*, 2008, 103:1562–1571.

49. *The International Tobacco Control Policy Evaluation Project: Thailand.* Waterloo, ON, The International Tobacco Control Policy Evaluation Project, 2010 (http://www.itcproject.org/projects/thailand/thexecsummaryyouth07pdf, accessed 12 April 2011).

50. Brown A, Moodie C. Adolescents' perceptions of tobacco control measures in the United Kingdom. *Health Promotion Practice*, 2010 (Epub ahead of print, 26 April).

51. Moodie C. Adolescents' response to text-only tobacco health warnings: results from the 2008 UK Youth Tobacco Policy Survey. *European Journal of Public Health*, 2010, 20:463–469.

52. Wade B et al. Cigarette pack warning labels in Russia: how graphic should they be? *European Journal of Public Health*, 2010 (Epub ahead of print, 21 July).

53. Abdullah AS. Predictors of women's attitudes toward World Health Organization Framework Convention on Tobacco Control policies in urban China. *Journal of Women's Health*, 2010, 19:903–909.

54. Yang T. Attitudes and behavioral response toward key tobacco control measures from the FCTC among Chinese urban residents. *BMC Public Health*, 2007, 7:248.

55. Wilson N et al. Distribution of new graphic warning labels: are tobacco companies following regulations? *Tobacco Induced Diseases*, 2009, 5:14.

56. Nakkash R, Khalil J. Health warning labelling practices on narghile (shisha, hookah) waterpipe tobacco products and related accessories. *Tobacco Control*, 2010, 19:235–239.

57. Roskin J et al. Canadian and English students' beliefs about waterpipe smoking: a qualitative study. *BMC Public Health*, 2009, 9:10.

58. Nakkash R et al. The tobacco industry's thwarting of marketing restrictions and health warnings in Lebanon. *Tobacco Control*, 2009, 18:310–316.

59. Oswal KC et al. Tobacco industry interference for pictorial warnings. *Indian Journal of Cancer*, 2010, 47(Suppl. 1):101–104.

60. Chapman S et al. "Avoid health warnings on all tobacco products for just as long as we can": a history of Australian tobacco industry efforts to avoid, delay and dilute health warnings on cigarettes. *Tobacco Control*, 2003, 12(Suppl. 3):iii13–iii22.

61. *Warning labels: countering industry arguments.* Washington, DC, Campaign for Tobacco-Free Kids, 2011 (http://www.tobaccofreecenter.org/files/pdfs/en/WL_industry_arguments_en.pdf, accessed 12 April 2011).

62. Davidson H. *"Cheeky buggers": Big Tobacco aims to get smokers angry about taxes, bans.* Surry Hills, NSW, News Limited, 1 April 2011 (http://www.news.com.au/national/cheeky-buggers-big tobacco launch campaign-against-anti-smoking-policies/story-e6frfkvr-1226031535298, accessed 12 April 2011).

63. Brinn MP et al. Mass media interventions for preventing smoking in young people. *Cochrane Database of Systematic Reviews*, 2010 (11):CD001006.

64. *Basic principles of media advocacy.* Geneva, World Health Organization, 2004 (http://www.who.int/tobacco/policy/media/en, accessed 12 April 2011).

65. *Applicability of the Fairness Doctrine to cigarette advertising.* Washington, DC, Federal Communications Commission, 1967 (32 Fed Reg 13162, 15 September 1967; http://tobaccodocuments.org/rjr/501881916-1928.html, accessed 12 April 2011).

66. Siegel M. Mass media antismoking campaigns: a powerful tool for health promotion. *Annals of Internal Medicine*, 1998, 129:128–132.

67. *Reducing tobacco use: a report of the Surgeon General.* Atlanta, GA, US Department of Health and Human Services, Centers for Disease Control and Prevention, National Centers for Chronic Disease Prevention and Health Promotion, Office on Smoking and Health, 2000.

68. Chan S. Health Dept. distributes matchbooks with grim alert. *The New York Times*, 22 Sept 2008:B3.

69. Ratcliffe J et al. Cost effectiveness of a mass media-led anti-smoking campaign in Scotland. *Tobacco Control*, 1997, 6:104–110.

70. *Best practices for comprehensive Tobacco Control Programs.* Atlanta, GA, US Department of Health and Human Services, Centers for Disease Control and Prevention, National Center for Chronic Disease Prevention and Health Promotion, Office on Smoking and Health, 2007 (http://www.cdc.gov/tobacco/stateandcommunity/best_practices/pdfs/2007/bestpractices_complete.pdf, accessed 12 April 2011).

71. Centers for Disease Control and Prevention (CDC). Decline in smoking prevalence – New York City, 2002–2006. *Morbidity and Mortality Weekly Report*, 2007, 56:604–608.

72. Frieden TR et al. Adult tobacco use levels after intensive tobacco control measures: New York City, 2002–2003. *American Journal of Public Health* 2005; 95:1016–1023.

73. Thrasher JF et al. Evaluation of a social marketing campaign to support Mexico City's comprehensive smoke-free law. *American Journal of Public Health*, 2011, 101:328–335.

74. Alday J et al. Smoke-free São Paulo: a campaign evaluation and the case for sustained mass media investment. *Salud Pública de México*, 2010, 52(Suppl. 2):S216–S225.

75. Murukutla M et al. Results of a national mass media campaign in India to warn against the dangers of smokeless tobacco consumption. *Tobacco Control*, 2011 (e-pub ahead of print, 20 Apr).

76. Gilpin EA at al. *Tobacco control successes in California: a focus on young people. Results from the California Tobacco Surveys, 1990–2002. Final Report.* La Jolla, CA, University of California, San Diego, 2003.

77. Biener L et al. *Massachusetts Adult Tobacco Survey: tobacco use and attitudes after seven years of the Massachusetts Tobacco Control Program. Technical Report and Tables 1993–2000.* Boston, MA, University of Massachusetts, Center for Survey Research, 2001.

78. Durkin S, Wakefield M. Comparative responses to radio and television anti-smoking advertisements to encourage smoking cessation. *Health Promotion International*, 2010, 25:5–13.

79. McVey D, Stapleton J. Can anti-smoking television advertising affect smoking behaviour? Controlled trial of the Health Education Authority for England's anti-smoking TV campaign. *Tobacco Control*, 2000, 9:273–282.

80. Siegel M, Biener L. The impact of an antismoking media campaign on progression to established smoking: results of a longitudinal youth study. *American Journal of Public Health*, 2000, 90:380–386.

81. Bala M et al. Mass media interventions for smoking cessation in adults. *Cochrane Database of Systematic Reviews*, 2008, (1) CD004704.

82. Wakefield MA et al. Impact of tobacco control policies and mass media campaigns on monthly adult smoking prevalence. *American Journal of Public Health*, 2008, 98:1443–1450.

83. Farrelly MC et al. The influence of the national Truth campaign on smoking initiation. *American Journal of Preventive Medicine*, 2009, 36:379–384.

84. Farrelly MC et al. Evidence of a dose-response relationship between "truth" antismoking ads and youth smoking prevalence. *American Journal of Public Health*, 2005, 95:425–431.

85. Cotter T et al. Smokers respond to anti-tobacco mass media campaigns in NSW by calling the Quitline. *NSW Public Health Bulletin*, 2008, 19:68–71.

86. Hyland A et al. Anti-tobacco television advertising and indicators of smoking cessation in adults: a cohort study. *Health Education Research*, 2006, 21:348–354.

87. Farrelly MC. Sustaining "truth": changes in youth tobacco attitudes and smoking intentions after 3 years of a national antismoking campaign. *Health Education Research*, 2009, 24:42–48.

88. Sly DF et al. Evidence of the dose effects of an antitobacco counteradvertising campaign. *Preventive Medicine*, 2002, 35:511–518.

89. Emery S et al. Televised state-sponsored antitobacco advertising and youth smoking beliefs and behavior in the United States, 1999–2000. *Archives of Pediatric and Adolescent Medicine*, 2005, 159:639–645.

90. *The Global Adult Tobacco Survey*. Atlanta, GA, Centers for Disease Control and Prevention, 2009 (http://www.cdc.gov/tobacco/global/gats/introduction/index.htm, accessed 19 April 2011).

91. Buller DB et al. Randomized trials on consider this, a tailored, internet-delivered smoking prevention program for adolescents. *Health and Education Behavior*, 2008, 35:260–281.

92. Abroms LC et al. iPhone apps for smoking cessation: a content analysis. *American Journal of Preventive Medicine*, 2011, 40:279–285.

93. Dunlop SM et al. The contribution of antismoking advertising to quitting: intra- and interpersonal processes. *Journal of Health Communication*, 2008, 13:250–266.

94. Leshner G et al. Scare 'em or disgust 'em: the effects of graphic health promotion messages. *Health Communication*, 2009, 24:447–458.

95. Davis KC et al. Exploring differences in smokers' perceptions of the effectiveness of cessation media messages. *Tobacco Control*, 2010, 20: 26–33.

96. Wakefield M et al. Comparison of the National Tobacco Campaign with a youth targeted South Australian campaign. In: Hassard K, ed. *Australia's National Tobacco Campaign: Evaluation report Volume one. Every cigarette is doing you damage*. Canberra, Commonwealth Department of Health and Aged Care, 1999; 255–268.

97. White VN et al. Do adult-focused anti-smoking campaigns have an impact on adolescents? The case of the Australian National Campaign. *Tobacco Control*, 2003, 12(Suppl. 2):ii23–ii29.

98. Dietz NA et al. The reach of a youth-oriented anti-tobacco media campaign on adult smokers. *Drug and Alcohol Dependence*, 2008, 93:180–184.

99. Vardavas CI et al. What defines an effective anti-tobacco TV advertisement? A pilot study among Greek adolescents. *International Journal of Environmental Research and Public Health*, 2010, 7:78–88.

100. Sutfin EL et al. Adolescents' responses to anti-tobacco advertising: exploring the role of adolescents' smoking status and advertisement theme. *Journal of Health Communication*, 2008, 13:480–500.

101. Biener L. Anti-tobacco advertisements by Massachusetts and Philip Morris: what teenagers think. *Tobacco Control*, 2002, 11(Suppl. 2):ii43–ii46.

102. Goldman LK, Glantz SA. Evaluation of antismoking advertising campaigns. *Journal of the American Medical Association*, 1998, 279:772–777.

103. Thrasher JF et al. Using anti-tobacco industry messages to prevent smoking among high-risk adolescents. *Health Education Research*, 2006, 21:325–337.

104. Biener L et al. How broadcast volume and emotional content affect youth recall of anti-tobacco advertising. *American Journal of Preventive Medicine*, 2008, 35:14–19.

105. Biener L et al. Adults' response to Massachusetts anti-tobacco television advertisements: impact of viewer and advertisement characteristics. *Tobacco Control*, 2000, 9:401–407.

106. Biener L et al. Impact of smoking cessation aids and mass media among recent quitters. *American Journal of Preventive Medicine*, 2006, 30:217–224.

107. *Tobacco use among US racial/ethnic minority groups: a report of the Surgeon General*. Atlanta, GA, US Department of Health and Human Services, Centers for Disease Control and Prevention, National Center for Chronic Disease Prevention and Health Promotion, Office on Smoking and Health, 1998 (http://www.cdc.gov/tobacco/data_statistics/sgr/sgr_1998/index.htm, accessed 12 April 2011).

108. Farrelly MC et al. Exploring the role of message sensation value in designing effective tobacco countermarketing advertisements. Paper presented at the World Conference on Tobacco OR Health, Helsinki, 2003.

109. Wakefield MR et al. Appraisal of antismoking advertising by youth at risk for regular smoking: a comparative study in the United States, Australia, and Britain. *Tobacco Control*, 2003, 12(Suppl. 2):ii82–ii86.

110. Terry-McElrath Y et al. The effect of antismoking advertisement executional characteristics on youth comprehension, appraisal, recall, and engagement. *Journal of Health Communication*, 2005, 10:124–143.

111. Czarnecki KD. Media campaign effectiveness in promoting a smoking-cessation program. *American Journal of Preventive Medicine*, 2010, 38(Suppl. 3):S333–S342.

112. Frieden TR et al. Public health in New York City, 2002–2007: confronting epidemics of the modern era. *International Journal of Epidemiology*, 2008, 37:966–977.

113. Siahpush M et al. Antismoking television advertising and socioeconomic variations in calls to Quitline. *Journal of Epidemiology and Community Health*, 2007, 61:298–301.

114. Cotter T et al. The case for recycling and adapting anti-tobacco mass media campaigns. *Tobacco Control*, 2010, 19:514–517.

115. Hamilton JL. The demand for cigarettes: advertising, the health scare, and the cigarette advertising ban. *Review of Economics and Statistics*, 1972, 54:401–411.

116. Warner KE. The effects of the anti-smoking campaign on cigarette consumption. *American Journal of Public Health*, 1977, 67:645–650.

117. Warner KE. Cigarette smoking in the 1970s: the impact o the antismoking campaign on consumption. *Science*, 198 211:729–731.

118. Hornik RC. Public health communication: making sense of contradictory evidence. In: Hornik RC, ed. *Public health communication: evidence for behavior change*. Mahwah, NJ, Lawrence Erlbaum, 2002:1–20.

119. McLeod J et al. On understanding and misunderstanding media effects. In: Curran J, Gurevitch M, eds. *Mass media and society*. London, Edward Arnold, 1991:235–266.

120. Schar E et al. *Tobacco use prevention media campaigns: lessons learned from youth in nine countries*. Atlanta, GA US Department of Health and Human Services, Centers for Disease Control and Prevention, National Center for Chronic Disease Prevention and Health Promotion, Office on Smoking and Health, 2006.

121. Hersey JC et al. How state counter-industry campaigns he prime perceptions of tobacco industry practices to promo reductions in youth smoking. *Tobacco Control*, 2005, 14:377–383.

122. Niederdeppe J et al. Consequences of dramatic reduction in state tobacco control funds: Florida, 1998–2000. *Tobac Control*, 2008, 17:205–210.

123. Dietz NA et al. Changes in youth cigarette use following the dismantling of an antitobacco media campaign in Florida. *Preventing Chronic Disease*, 2010, 7:A65.

124. Centers for Disease Control and Prevention (CDC). Effect of ending an antitobacco youth campaign on adolescent susceptibility to cigarette smoking – Minnesota, 2002–2003. *Morbidity and Mortality Weekly Report*, 200 53:301–304.

125. Hafstad A et al. Provocative appeals in anti-smoking mas media campaigns targeting adolescents – the accumulate effect of multiple exposures. *Health Education Research*, 1997, 12:227–236.

126. *Tobacco control mass media resource*. New York, NY, World Lung Foundation, 2010 (http://67.199.72.89/mmr/english/360mmrProcess.html, accessed 12 April 2011).

127. Smith EA, Malone RE. Philip Morris's health information web site appears responsible but undermines public heal *Public Health Nursing*, 2008, 25:554–564.

128. Sebrié EM, Glantz SA. Attempts to undermine tobacco control: tobacco industry "youth smoking prevention" programs to undermine meaningful tobacco control in Latin America. *American Journal of Public Health*, 2007, 97:1357–1367.

129. Wakefield M et al. Effect of televised, tobacco company-funded smoking prevention advertising on youth smoking related beliefs, intentions, and behavior. *American Journa of Public Health*, 2006, 96:2154–2160.

130. Farrelly MC et al. Getting to the truth: evaluating national tobacco countermarketing campaigns. *American Journal Public Health*, 2002, 92:901–907.

131. Henriksen LA et al. Industry-sponsored anti-smoking ads and adolescent reactance: test of a boomerang effect. *Tobacco Control*, 2006, 15:13–18.

132. Healton C. Who's afraid of the truth? *American Journal of Public Health*, 2001, 91:554–558.

133. *Guidelines for implementation of Article 5.3 of the WHO Framework Convention on Tobacco Control (Protection of public health policies with respect to tobacco control from commercial and other vested interests of the tobacco industry)*. Geneva, World Health Organization, 2008 (http://www.who.int/fctc/guidelines/article_5_3/en/index.html, accessed 25 May 2011).

134. *Enforcing strong smokefree laws: the advocate's guide to enforcement strategies*. Atlanta, GA, American Cancer Society, 2006 (American Cancer Society/UICC Tobacco Control Strategy Planning Guide #4).

135. Wolfson M. *The fight against big tobacco: the movement, the state, and the public's health*. New York, NY, Aldine Transaction, 2001.

136. Chapman S, Dominello A. A strategy for increasing news media coverage of tobacco and health in Australia. *Health Promotion International*, 2001, 16:137–143.

137. Laugesen M, Meads C. Advertising, price, income and publicity effects on weekly cigarette sales in New Zealand supermarkets. *British Journal of Addiction*, 1991, 86:83–89.

138. Cummings KM et al. Impact of a newspaper mediated quit smoking program. *American Journal of Public Health*, 1987, 77:1452–1453.

139. Pierce JP, Gilpin EA. News media coverage of smoking and health is associated with changes in population rates of smoking cessation but not initiation. *Tobacco Control*, 2001, 10:145–153.

140. Smith KC et al. Relationship between newspaper coverage of tobacco issues and perceived smoking harm and smoking behaviour among American teens. *Tobacco Control*, 2008, 17:17–24.

141. McGoldrick DE, Boonn AV. Public policy to maximize tobacco cessation. *American Journal of Preventive Medicine*, 2010, 38(Suppl. 3):S327–S332.

142. *WHO report on the global tobacco epidemic, 2008: the MPOWER package*. Geneva, World Health Organization, 2008 (http://www.who.int/tobacco/mpower/gtcr_download/en/index.html, accessed 12 April 2011).

143. *WHO report on the global tobacco epidemic, 2009: implementing smoke-free environments*. Geneva, World Health Organization, 2009 (http://www.who.int/tobacco/mpower/2009/en/index.html, accessed 12 April 2011).

144. *Philippines (ages 13–15) Global Youth Tobacco Survey (GYTS) Fact Sheets*. Data retrieved from Global Tobacco Surveillance System Data (GTSSData). Atlanta, GA, Centers for Disease Control and Prevention (http://apps.nccd.cdc.gov/GTSSData/Ancillary/DataReports.aspx?Option=1, accessed 12 April 2011).

145. Miguel-Baquilod M. *Piloting of the Global Health Professionals Tobacco Survey (GHPS) among pharmacy school students in the Philippines*. Manila, Department of Health, 2005 (http://www.wpro.who.int/NR/rdonlyres/1A3DF538-0143-4B89-8488-C22008E9A1DE/0/PHLGHPS2005.pdf, accessed 12 April 2011).

146. *2009 Philippines' Global Adult Tobacco Survey Country Report*. Geneva, World Health Organization, 2010 (http://www.who.int/tobacco/surveillance/2009_gats_report_philippines.pdf, accessed 12 April 2011).

147. *Guidelines for implementation of Article 8 of the WHO Framework Convention on Tobacco Control (Protection from exposure to tobacco smoke)*. Geneva, World Health Organization, 2007 (http://www.who.int/fctc/guidelines/article_8/en/index.html, accessed 25 May 2011).

148. *Smoke-free air: the essential facts*. Washington, DC, Campaign for Tobacco-Free Kids, 2007 (http://tobaccofreecenter.org/files/pdfs/en/SF_facts_en.pdf, accessed 12 April 2011).

149. *Evaluating the effectiveness of smoke-free policies*. Lyon, International Agency for Research on Cancer, 2009 (IARC Handbooks of Cancer Prevention, Tobacco Control, Vol. 13: http://www.iarc.fr/en/publications/pdfs-online/prev/handbook13/index.php, accessed 25 May 2011).

150. *How tobacco smoke causes disease: the biology and behavioral basis for smoking-attributable disease. A report of the Surgeon General*. Atlanta, GA, US Department of Health and Human Services, Centers for Disease Control and Prevention, National Center for Chronic Disease Prevention and Health Promotion, Office on Smoking and Health, 2010 (http://www.surgeongeneral.gov/library/tobaccosmoke/report/full_report.pdf, accessed 12 April 2011).

151. *Secondhand smoke exposure and cardiovascular effects: making sense of the evidence*. Washington, DC, Institute of Medicine, National Academies Press, 2009.

152. Viswanathan B et al. Impact of a smoking ban in public places: a rapid assessment in the Seychelles. *Tobacco Control*, 2011 (Epub ahead of print, 28 March).

153. *Guidelines for implementation of Article 14 of the WHO Framework Convention on Tobacco Control (Demand reduction measures concerning tobacco dependence and cessation)*. Geneva, World Health Organization, 2010 (http://www.who.int/fctc/guidelines/article_14/en/index.html, accessed 25 May 2011).

154. Fiore MC et al. *Treating tobacco use and dependence*. Hyattsville, MD, US Department of Health and Human Services, Public Health Service, 2008 (Clinical Practice Guideline. 2008 update).

155. Shanghai World Expo ditches 200-mln yuan tobacco sponsorship. Beijing, *People's Daily Online*, 22 July 2009 (http://english.peopledaily.com.cn/90001/90776/90882/6707290.html, accessed 12 April 2011).

156. *The 16th Asian Games to be tobacco-free*. Beijing, Chinese Olympic Committee, 2009 (http://en.olympic.cn/news/olympic_news/2009-11-20/1925365.html, accessed 12 April 2011).

157. *Kelly Clarkson dumps Indonesia tobacco sponsor*. New York, NY, Associated Press, 22 April 2010 (http://www.cbsnews.com/stories/2010/04/22/entertainment/main6421011.shtml, accessed 12 April 2011).

158. *WHO technical manual on tobacco tax administration*. Geneva, World Health Organization, 2010 (http://www.who.int/tobacco/publications/tax_administration/en/index.html, accessed 12 April 2011).

159. *Conference of the Parties to the WHO Framework Convention on Tobacco Control, fourth session. Decisions*. Geneva, WHO Framework Convention on Tobacco Control, 2010 (FCTC/COP/4/DIV/6; http://www.who.int/fctc/copdecisionrevone.pdf, accessed 12 April 2010).

160. *Increasing tobacco taxation revenue in Egypt*. Geneva, World Health Organization, 2010 (http://www.emro.who.int/tfi/PDF/FactsheetEgypt2010.pdf, accessed 12 April 2010).

161. David A, Esson K, Perucic A-M, Fitzpatrick C. Tobacco use: equity and social determinants. In: Blas E, Sivasankara Kurup A, eds. *Equity, Social Determinants and Public Health Programmes*. Geneva, World Health Organization, 2010.

162. *Concept of creation of a public policy on combating tobacco consumption from 2010–2015*. Moscow, Government of the Russian Federation, 23 September 2010 (http://www.tobaccofreecenter.org/files/pdfs/en/Russian_Concept_on_Tobacco_en.pdf, accessed 12 April 2011).

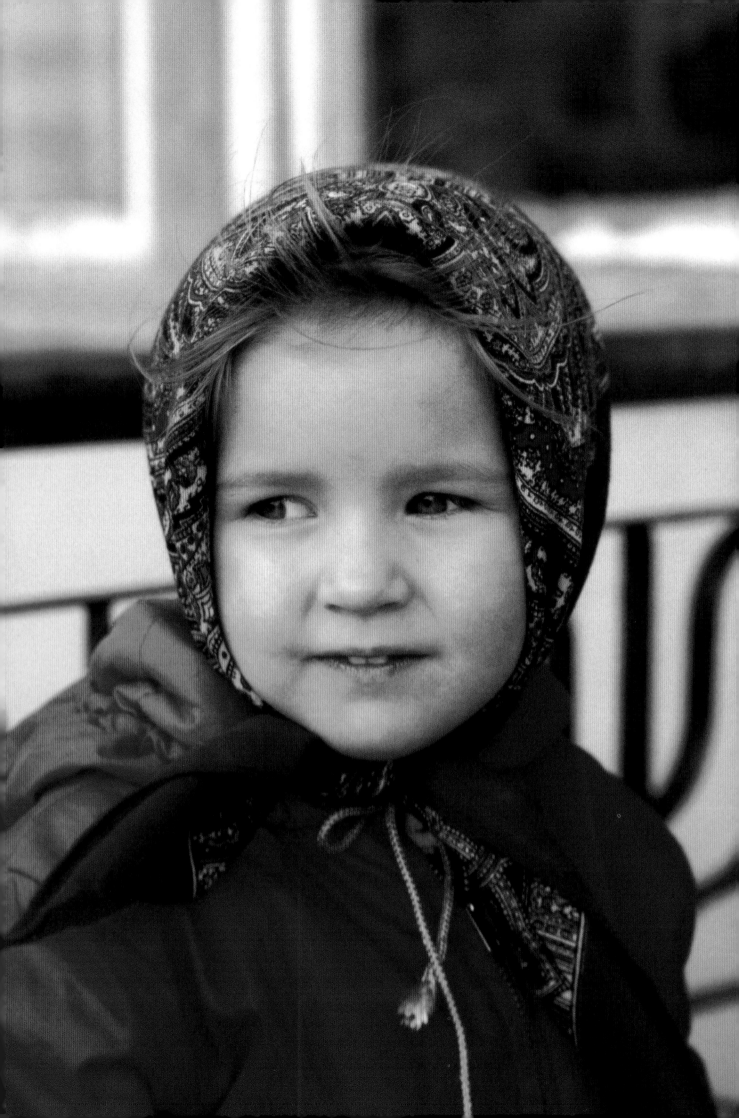

TECHNICAL NOTES

APPENDICES

Appendices IV through X are available in electronic format on the CD
on page 155 of this book and online at http://www.who.int/tobacco/

TECHNICAL NOTE I
Evaluation of existing policies and compliance

To ensure consistency and comparability among *WHO Reports on the Global Tobacco Epidemic, 2008* and *2009* and this report, the data collection and analysis methodology used are based largely on previous reports. Some of the methodology employed in earlier reports has been revised and strengthened for the present report. Where revisions have been made, data from previous reports have been reanalysed so that the results are comparable across years. The methodology employed for this year's report is described in this Technical Note.

Data sources

Data were collected using the following sources:

- For all areas: official reports from WHO FCTC Parties to the Conference of the Parties (COP), through the Convention Secretariat[1].
- For M: tobacco prevalence surveys not yet reported under the COP reporting mechanism were collected from the WHO Global Infobase and through an extensive literature search. Technical Note II provides the detailed methodology used.
- For P, W (pack warnings) and E: original tobacco control legislation adopted in all Member States related to smoke-free environments, comprehensive bans on tobacco advertising, promotion and sponsorship, and packaging and labelling measures were carefully reviewed, as described below.
- For W (mass media): data on anti-tobacco mass media campaigns were obtained from Member States. In order to avoid unnecessary data collection, the Tobacco Free Initiative conducted a screening for anti-tobacco mass media campaigns in all WHO country offices. In countries where potentially eligible mass media campaigns were identified, focal points in each country were contacted for further information on these campaigns.
- For R: the prices of the most sold brand of cigarettes, the cheapest brand and the brand Marlboro were collected for July 2010 through regional data collectors. The information on the taxation of cigarettes (and, for some countries in SEAR, bidis) and revenues from tobacco taxation as well as any supporting documents were collected from ministries of finance. Technical Note III provides the detailed methodology used.

Based on these sources of information, WHO ascertained the value of each of the 131 variables used for the report as of 31 December 2010, except for monitoring surveys of tobacco use, which were appraised as of November 2010, tobacco product prices and taxes, which were appraised as of July 2010, and anti-tobacco media campaigns, which were appraised as of August 2010.

Data validation

For each country, each data point was assessed independently by two different expert staff from two different WHO offices, generally one from WHO headquarters and the other from the respective regional office. Any inconsistencies found were reviewed by the two WHO expert staff involved and a third expert staff member not yet involved in the appraisal of the legislation and were resolved by: (i) checking the original text of the legislation; (ii) trying to obtain consensus from the two expert staff involved in the data collection; and (iii) in case differences still remained, decision of the third expert. Data were also checked for completeness and logical consistency across variables.

Data sign-off

The final validated data for each country were sent to the respective government for review and sign-off. To facilitate review by governments, a summary sheet was generated for each country and was sent for review prior to the close of the report database. In cases where national authorities explicitly did not approve any of the data, this is specifically noted in the appendix tables.

Further details about the data processing procedure are available from the WHO Tobacco Free Initiative.

Data analysis

The report provides summary measures or indicators of country achievements for each of the six MPOWER measures. The summary measures developed for the *WHO Report on the Global Tobacco Epidemic, 2011* are the same as those used for the 2009 report, except for the indicator on health warnings, which was slightly improved and the indicator on anti-tobacco mass media campaigns, which is new. These two measures

constitute the central topic of the present report. It is important to note that data for the report are based on existing legislation and reflect the status of adopted but not necessarily implemented legislation, as long as the law clearly indicates a date of entry into force and is not undergoing a legal challenge.

When country or population totals for MPOWER measures are referred to collectively in the analysis section of this report, only the implementation of tobacco control policies (smoke-free legislation, cessation services, warning labels, anti-tobacco mass media campaigns, advertising and promotion bans, and tobacco taxes) is included in these totals. Monitoring of tobacco use is reported separately. When changes in population coverage since 2008 are presented, again only implementation of policies is included, except for data on implementation of anti-tobacco mass media campaigns; since these data were collected for the first time in 2010 and thus no comparative data are available for 2008.

Correction to previously published data

The data from the 2009 edition of the report were reviewed, and about 3% of data points were corrected. In most cases, review was conducted because legislation was in place at the time of the 2009 report but not available to WHO in time for publication[2]. As a result of these corrections four countries were downgraded from the highest group of smoke-free legislation, one country for cessation services, ten countries for bans on advertising, promotion and sponsorship, and two countries for tax rates.

Monitoring

The section of the report devoted to assessing each country's achievements in monitoring notes the most recent smoking prevalence survey data available and includes the following information:

- the recentness of the survey;
- whether the survey was representative of the country's population;
- whether it covered adults, youth or both;
- whether the survey was repeated at least every five years (survey periodicity).

Surveys were considered recent if the data were

collected in 2005 or later. Surveys were considered representative if the sample was representative of the national population. Surveys were considered periodic if they were conducted at least once every five years. Surveys were considered "adult surveys" if participants were above 15 years of age. Surveys were considered "youth surveys" if all participants were between 11 and 19 years of age. For this year's report, the groupings for the Monitoring indicator have been revised to reflect the additional information collected on survey periodicity. Periodicity of surveys of at least every five years is included in the highest category in addition to the requirements of recent and representative data for both adults and youth. Because of this, some countries that fell in the highest category in the previous report (defined as those having recent and representative data only) do not fall in the highest category in this report. The groupings for the Monitoring indicator are listed below.

	No known data or no recent* data or data that are not both recent* and not representative**
	Recent* and representative** data for either adults or youth
	Recent* and representative** data for both adults and youth
	Recent*, representative** and periodic*** data for both adults and youth

* Data from 2005 or later.
** Survey sample representative of the national population.
*** Occurring at least every five years.

Smoke-free legislation

There is a wide range of places and institutions which can be made smoke-free by law. Smoke-free legislation can take place at the national or subnational level. The report includes data on national legislation as well as legislation in subnational jurisdictions. The assessment of subnational smoke-free legislation includes all first-level administrative boundaries (first administrative subdivisions of a country), as determined by the United Nations Geographical Information Working Group (UNGIWG). In addition, smoke-free legislation status of other subnational jurisdictions is reported when data and respective legislation were provided by country focal points. Legislation was assessed to determine whether smoke-free laws at either the national or subnational level provided for a complete[3] indoor smoke-free environment at all

times, in all the facilities of each of the following places:

- health-care facilities;
- educational facilities other than universities;
- universities;
- government facilities;
- indoor offices and workplaces not considered in any other category;
- restaurants or facilities that serve mostly food;
- pubs and bars or facilities that serve mostly beverages (not applicable where alcohol serving is illegal);
- public transport.

Groupings for the Smoke-free legislation indicator are based on the numbers of places and institutions where smoking is completely prohibited. In addition, countries where at least 90% of the population was covered by complete subnational indoor smoke-free legislation are grouped in the top category.

In a few countries, in order to significantly expand the creation of smoke-free places, including restaurants and bars, it was politically necessary to include exceptions to the law that allowed for the provision of designated smoking rooms (DSRs) with requirements so technically complex and strict that, for practical purposes, few or no establishments are expected to implement them. In order to meet the criteria for "very strict technical requirements", the legislation had to include at least three out of the six following characteristics (and must include at least criteria #5 or #6).

The designated smoking room must:

1. be a closed indoor environment;
2. be furnished with automatic doors, generally kept closed;
3. be non-transit premises for non-smokers;
4. be furnished with appropriate forced-ventilation mechanical devices;
5. have appropriate installations and functional openings installed and air must be expelled from the premises;
6. be maintained, with reference to surrounding areas, in a depression not lower than 5 Pascal.

The five countries meeting these criteria have not been categorized in the analyses for this section because their smoke-free legislation substantially departs from the recommendations of WHO FCTC Article 8 guidelines, and it has been difficult to obtain evidence indicating that the law resulted in the intended very low number of DSRs in all of these countries.

The groupings for the Smoke-free legislation indicator are listed below.

	Data not reported/not categorized
	Up to two public places completely smoke-free
	Three to five public places completely smoke-free
	Six to seven public places completely smoke-free
	All public places* completely smoke-free (or at least 90% of the population covered by complete subnational smoke-free legislation)

* In a country where pubs and bars are illegal, only seven places are required to be smoke-free to qualify for this group.

Tobacco dependence treatment

Despite the low cost of quit lines, few low- or middle-income countries have implemented such programmes. Thus, national toll-free quit lines are included as a qualification only for the highest category. Reimbursement for tobacco dependence treatment is considered only for the top two categories to take restricted national budgets of many lower-income countries into consideration. The top three categories reflect varying levels of government commitment to the availability of nicotine replacement therapy and cessation support.

The groupings for the Tobacco dependence treatment indicator are listed below.

	Data not reported
	None
	NRT* and/or some cessation services** (neither cost-covered)
	NRT* and/or some cessation services** (at least one of which is cost-covered)
	National quit line, and both NRT* and some cessation services** cost-covered

* Nicotine replacement therapy.
** Smoking cessation support available in any of the following places: health clinics or other primary care facilities, hospitals, office of a health professional, the community.

Warning labels

The section of the report devoted to assessing each country's achievements in health warnings notes the following information about cigarette pack warnings:

- whether specific health warnings are mandated;
- the mandated size of the warnings, as a percentage of the front and back of the cigarette pack;

- whether the warnings appear on individual packages as well as on any outside packaging and labelling used in retail sale;
- whether the warnings describe specific harmful effects of tobacco use on health;
- whether the warnings are large, clear, visible and legible (e.g. specific colours and font styles and sizes are mandated);
- whether the warnings rotate;
- whether the warnings are written in (all) the principal language(s) of the country;
- whether the warnings include pictures or pictograms.

The size of the warnings on both the front and back of the cigarette pack were averaged to calculate the percentage of the total pack surface area that is covered by the warnings. This information was combined with the warning characteristics to construct the groupings for the Health warnings indicator.

The groupings for the Health warnings indicator are listed below.

	Data not reported
	No warnings or small warnings[1]
	Medium size warnings[2] missing some[3] appropriate characteristics[4] OR large warnings[5] missing many[6] appropriate characteristics[4]
	Medium size warnings[2] with all appropriate characteristics[4] OR large warnings[5] missing some[3] appropriate characteristics[4]
	Large warnings[5] with all appropriate characteristics[4]

[1] Average of front and back of package is less than 30%.
[2] Average of front and back of package is between 30 and 49%.
[3] One or more.
[4] Appropriate characteristics:
  - specific health warnings mandated;
  - appearing on individual packages as well as on any outside packaging and labelling used in retail sale;
  - describing specific harmful effects of tobacco use on health;
  - are large, clear, visible and legible (e.g. specific colours and font style and sizes are mandated);
  - rotate;
  - include pictures or pictograms;
  - written in (all) the principal language(s) of the country.
[5] Average of front and back of the package is at least 50%.
[6] Four or more.

Anti-tobacco mass media campaigns

There is a wide range of anti-tobacco mass media campaigns that are implemented in many countries each year. In order to focus the reporting on mass media campaigns that are likely to change attitudes about tobacco use, curb smoking initiation and encourage cessation, only those campaigns that had a duration of at least three weeks and were implemented at the national level between January 2009 and August 2010 were assessed for this report.

Eligible campaigns were assessed by the following characteristics:

- the campaign was part of a comprehensive tobacco control programme;
- before the campaign, research was undertaken or reviewed to gain a thorough understanding of the target audience;
- campaign communications materials were pre-tested with the target audience and refined in line with campaign objectives;
- air time (radio, television) and/or placement (billboards, print advertising, etc.) was obtained by purchasing or securing it using either the organization's own internal resources or an external media planner or agency (this information indicates whether the campaign adopted a thorough media planning and buying process to effectively and efficiently reach its target audience);
- the implementing agency worked with journalists to gain publicity or news coverage for the campaign;
- process evaluation was undertaken to assess how effectively the campaign had been implemented;
- an outcome evaluation process was implemented to assess the campaign impact.

The groupings for the Mass media campaigns indicator are listed below.

	Data not reported
	No campaign conducted between January 2009 and August 2010 with a duration of at least three weeks
	Campaign conducted with one to four appropriate characteristics
	Campaign conducted with five to six appropriate characteristics
	Campaign conducted with all appropriate characteristics

Bans on advertising, promotion and sponsorship

Country-level achievements in banning tobacco advertising, promotion and sponsorship were assessed based on whether the bans covered the following types of advertising:

- national television and radio;
- local magazines and newspapers;
- billboards and outdoor advertising;
- point of sale;
- free distribution of tobacco products in the mail or through other means;
- promotional discounts;
- non-tobacco goods and services identified with tobacco brand names (brand extension);
- brand names of non-tobacco products used for tobacco products[3];
- appearance of tobacco products in television and/or films;
- sponsored events.

The first four bans listed are considered "direct" advertising bans, and the remaining six are considered "indirect" bans. Complete bans on tobacco advertising, promotion and sponsorship usually start with bans on direct advertising in national media and progress to bans on indirect advertising as well as promotion and sponsorship. Bans that cover national television, radio and print media were used as the basic criteria for the two lowest groups, and the remaining groups were constructed based on how comprehensively the law covers the forms of direct and indirect bans included in the questionnaire.

The groupings for the Bans on advertising, promotion and sponsorship indicator are listed below.

	Data not reported
	Complete absence of ban, or ban that does not cover national television (TV), radio and print media
	Ban on national TV, radio and print media only
	Ban on national TV, radio and print media as well as on some but not all other forms of direct* and/or indirect** advertising
	Ban on all forms of direct* and indirect** advertising

* Direct advertising bans:
  - national television and radio;
  - local magazines and newspapers;
  - billboards and outdoor advertising;
  - point of sale.
** Indirect advertising bans:
  - free distribution of tobacco products in the mail or through other means;
  - promotional discounts;
  - non-tobacco goods and services identified with tobacco brand names (brand extension);
  - brand names of non-tobacco products used for tobacco products;
  - appearance of tobacco products in television and/ or films;
  - sponsored events.

Tobacco taxes

Countries are grouped according to the percentage contribution of taxes to the retail price. Taxes assessed include excise tax, value added tax (sometimes called "VAT"), import duty (when the cigarettes were imported) and any other taxes levied. Only the price of the most popular brand of cigarettes is considered. In the case of countries where different levels of taxes are applied to cigarettes are based on either length, quantity produced or type (e.g. filter vs non-filter), only the rate that applied to the most popular brand is used in the calculation.

Given the lack of information on country and brand-specific profit margins of retailers and wholesalers, their profits were assumed to be zero (unless provided by the national data collector).

The groupings for the Tobacco tax indicator are listed below. Please refer to Technical Note III for more details.

	Data not reported
	≤ 25% of retail price is tax
	26–50% of retail price is tax
	51–75% of retail price is tax
	>75% of retail price is tax

National tobacco control programmes

Classification of countries' national tobacco control programmes is based on the existence of a national agency with responsibility for tobacco control objectives. Countries with at least five full-time equivalent staff members working at the national agency with responsibility for tobacco control meet the criteria for the highest group.

The groupings for the National tobacco control programme indicator are listed below.

	Data not reported
	No national agency on tobacco control
	Existence of national agency with responsibility for tobacco control objectives with no or < 5 full-time equivalent staff members
	Existence of national agency with responsibility for tobacco control objectives and at least 5 full-time equivalent staff members

Compliance assessment

Compliance with national and comprehensive subnational smoke-free legislation as well as with advertising, promotion and sponsorship bans

(covering both direct and indirect marketing) was assessed by up to five national experts, who assessed the compliance in these two areas as "minimal", "moderate" or "high". These five experts were selected according to the following criteria:

- person in charge of tobacco prevention in the country's ministry of health, or the most senior government official in charge of tobacco control or tobacco-related conditions;
- the head of a prominent nongovernmental organization dedicated to tobacco control;
- a health professional (e.g. physician, nurse, pharmacist or dentist) specializing in tobacco-related conditions;
- a staff member of a public health university department;
- the Tobacco Free Initiative focal point of the WHO country office.

The experts performed their assessments independently. Summary scores were calculated by WHO from the five individual assessments by assigning two points for highly enforced policies, one point for moderately enforced policies and no points for minimally enforced policies, with a potential minimum of 0 and maximum of 10 points in total from these five experts. The compliance assessment was obtained for legislation that had been adopted by 30 June 2010. For countries with more recent legislation, the compliance data are reported as *not applicable*.

To expedite the process of collecting compliance scores, compliance data for this report were collected differently than in previous years. For this report, where possible, the same experts were contacted directly by WHO regional staff and were asked to provide their assessment of compliance. Where this was not possible (because either there were no experts from the previous report(s) or the original experts could not be located), WHO regional and country offices made contact with other appropriate experts employing the same selection criteria described above. To assess possible bias in this report's compliance scores resulting from this change in procedure, experts' compliance assessments were compared for countries where the legislation on smoke-free legislation and advertising, promotion and sponsorship bans had not changed since the last report. Three quarters of eligible countries had the same or almost the same compliance scores as in the previous report, indicating that the different method of obtaining the compliance data did not result in significantly different values.

The country-reported answers are listed in Appendix IV. Appendix I summarizes this information. Compliance scores are represented separately (i.e. compliance is not included in the calculation of the grouping categories).

[1] Parties report on the implementation of the WHO Framework Convention on Tobacco Control according to Article 21. The objective of reporting is to enable Parties to learn from each other's experience in implementing the WHO FCTC. Parties' reports are also the basis for review by the COP of the implementation of the Convention. Parties submit their initial report two years after entry into force of the WHO FCTC for that Party, and then every subsequent three years, through the reporting instrument adopted by COP. Starting in 2012, all Parties will report at the same time, once every two years. For more information please refer to http://www.who.int/fctc/reporting/en/

[2] Further analysis found that information for a few countries had been misinterpreted in prior reports; for these countries, the response has been changed accordingly in this report.

[3] "Complete" is used in this report to mean that smoking is not permitted, with no exemptions allowed, except in residences and indoor places that serve as equivalents to long-term residential facilities, such as prisons and long-term health and social care facilities. Ventilation and any form of designated smoking rooms and/or areas do not protect from the harms of second-hand tobacco smoke, and the only laws that provide protection are those that result in the complete absence of smoking in all public places.

TECHNICAL NOTE II

Smoking prevalence in WHO Member States

Monitoring the prevalence of tobacco use is central to any surveillance system for tobacco control. Reliable prevalence data provide the information needed to assess the impacts of tobacco control actions adopted by a country and can be used by tobacco control workers in their efforts to counter the tobacco epidemic. This report contains WHO-modelled prevalence estimates for smoking and country-provided data for both smoking and smokeless tobacco use (see Appendix VII).

Collection of tobacco use prevalence estimates

As discussed in Technical Note I, the data collection process for this report differed from that used in the previous two editions of the *WHO Report on the Global Tobacco Epidemic*. Information for the previous reports was collected by sending a detailed questionnaire to Member States about any tobacco survey that had been conducted in the relatively recent past. For this report, three sources of data were first explored: (i) reports submitted to the WHO FCTC Secretariat by Parties; and (ii) information sought from the WHO STEPwise Survey team (also responsible for the WHO Global Infobase, a portal of information on eight risk factors for noncommunicable diseases including tobacco: http://www.who.int/infobase) on countries that may have conducted or officially released the results of a recent survey implemented since 2005. In addition, an extensive literature search was conducted to identify any other possible data sources. During this process, multiple data sources were frequently identified. In such cases, preference was given to surveys that met the following four criteria:

- provide country survey summary data for one or more of four tobacco use definitions: daily smoker, current smoker, daily cigarette smoker or current cigarette smoker;
- include randomly selected participants who were representative of a general population;
- present prevalence values by age and sex;

- survey the adult population aged 15 years and older.

Member States were contacted if WHO did not obtain an official report from the recently undertaken surveys.

Data were collated on four indicators of tobacco smoking:

- current and daily prevalence of tobacco smoking;[1]
- current and daily prevalence of cigarette smoking.

These indicators provide the most complete representation of tobacco smoking across countries. Although differences exist in the types of tobacco products used in different countries and grown or manufactured in different regions of the world, data on cigarette smoking and tobacco smoking are the most widely available and are common to all countries, thereby permitting statistical analyses.[2]

Analysis and presentation of tobacco use prevalence estimates

In this report, prevalence data are presented in two forms - crude rates provided directly by countries (Appendix VIII) and age-standardized rates for adults aged 15 years and over estimated by WHO (Appendix VII). To produce the age-standardized rates for the various indicators of tobacco and cigarette smoking described above for one common year (2009), WHO first adjusted the country-provided data for differences in survey methods including differences in age-groups, indicators of tobacco use, geographic coverage and survey year. After these adjustments were made, WHO then produced directly age-standardized estimates to enable cross-country comparisons.

Adjustments to country provided data

Data from various surveys undertaken in countries

provide an estimate of tobacco use. Typically, these estimates are provided as crude rates, expressed as the percentage of tobacco users of the total survey sample. These rates are useful to estimate the number of smokers for the relevant indicator (e.g. current smokers, daily smokers) in the population. If the surveys in countries used standard methods across time, then projecting crude tobacco estimates for one point in time (2009 for this report) would be a relatively simple task. However, many countries use a variety of survey sources that do not apply standardized survey instruments.

WHO has developed a regression method that attempts to adjust the estimates to enable comparisons of results between countries. The general principle that underlies the regression method is that if data are partly missing or are incomplete for a country, then the regression technique uses data available for the region in which the country is located to generate estimates for that country. The regression models are run at the United Nations subregional level[3] separately for males and females in order to obtain age-specific prevalence rates for that region. These estimates are then substituted for the country falling within the subregion for the missing indicator. Note that the technique cannot be used for countries without any data; these countries are excluded from any analysis. The four types of differences between surveys and the relevant adjustment procedures used are listed below.

Differences in age groups covered by the survey. In order to estimate smoking prevalence rates for standard age ranges (by five-year groups from age 15 until age 80 and then aggregated from 80 to 100 years), the association between age and daily smoking is examined for males and females separately for each country using scatter plots. For this exercise, data from the latest nationally representative survey are chosen; in some cases more than one survey is chosen if male and female prevalence rates stem from different surveys or if the additional survey supplements data for the extreme age intervals. To obtain age-specific prevalence rates for five-year age intervals, regression models using daily smoking prevalence estimates from a first-order, second-order and third-order function of age are graphed against the scatter plot and the best-fitting curve is chosen. For the remaining indicators, a combination of methods is applied: regression models are run at the subregional level to obtain age-specific rates for current and daily cigarette smoking, and an equivalence relationship is applied between smoking prevalence rates and cigarette smoking where cigarette smoking is dominant to obtain age-specific prevalence rates for current and daily cigarette smoking for the standard age intervals.

Differences in the types of indicators of tobacco use measured. If we have data for current tobacco smoking and current cigarette smoking, then definitional adjustments are made to account for the missing daily tobacco smoking and daily cigarette smoking data. Likewise, if we have data for current and daily tobacco smoking only, then tobacco type adjustments are made across tobacco types to generate estimates for current and daily cigarette smoking.

Differences in geographic coverage of the survey within the country. Adjustments are made to the data by observing the prevalence relationship between urban and rural areas in countries falling within the relevant subregion. Results from this urban-rural regression exercise are applied to countries to allow a scaling-up of prevalence to the national level. As an example, if a country has prevalence rates for daily smoking of tobacco in urban areas only, the regression results from the smoking relationship are used to obtain rural prevalence rates for daily smoking. These are then combined with urban prevalence rates using urban-rural population ratios as weights to generate a national prevalence estimate as well as national age-specific rates.

Differences in survey year. For this report, smoking prevalence estimates are generated for the year 2009. Smoking prevalence data are sourced from

surveys conducted in countries in different years. In some cases, the latest available prevalence data came from surveys before the year 2009 while in other cases the survey was later than 2009. To obtain smoking prevalence estimates for 2009, trend information is used either to project into the future for countries with data older than 2009 or backtracked for countries with data later than 2009. This is achieved by incorporating trend information from all available surveys for each country. For countries without historical data, trend information from the respective subregion in which they fall is used.

Estimation of number of smokers. Adjusted prevalence estimates can be used to assess the number of smokers for the relevant indicator in a country.

Estimation of age-standardized prevalence rates. Tobacco use generally varies widely by sex and across age groups. Although the adjusted prevalence rate is reasonably easy to understand for a country at one point in time, comparing prevalence rates between two or more countries at one point in time, or of one country at different points in time, can be misleading if the two populations being compared have significantly different age distributions or differences in tobacco use by sex. The method of age standardization is commonly used to overcome this problem and allows for meaningful comparison of prevalence between countries. The method involves applying the age-specific rates by sex in each population to one standard population. When presenting age-standardized prevalence rates, both this and the previous WHO reports on the global tobacco epidemic used the WHO Standard Population, a fictitious population whose age distribution was artificially created and is largely reflective of the population age structure of low- and middle-income countries. The resulting age-standardized rate, also expressed as a percentage of the total population, refers to the number of smokers per 100 WHO Standard Population. As a result, the rate generated using this process is only a

hypothetical number with no inherent meaning in itself. It is only useful when comparing rates obtained from one country with those obtained in another country, or from the same country at a different point in time. In order to produce an overall smoking prevalence rate for a country, the age-standardized prevalence rates for males and females must be combined to generate total prevalence. Since the WHO Standard Population is the same irrespective of sex, the age-standardized rates for males and females are combined using population weights for males and for females at the global level from United Nations population data for 2009. For example, if the age-standardized prevalence rate for tobacco smoking in adults is 60% for males and 30% for females, the combined prevalence rate for tobacco smoking in all adults is calculated as 60 x (0.51) + 30 x (0.49) = 45%, with the figures in brackets representing male and female population weights. Thus, of the total smoking prevalence (45%), the proportion of smoking attributable to males is 66.7% [= (30 ÷ 45) x 100] and to females 33.3% [= (15 ÷ 45) x 100]. These combined rates are shown in Appendix VII.

1 Tobacco smoking includes cigarettes, cigars, pipes and any other form of smoked tobacco.

2 For countries where consumption of smokeless tobacco products is high, we have published these data for that particular country.

3 There are 21 United Nations subregions; Oceania, Melanesia, Polynesia and Micronesia are combined into one subregion to form a total of 18. For a complete listing, please refer to World Population Prospects, 2008 revision at http://esa.un.org/unpp/index.asp?panel=5

TECHNICAL NOTE III

Tobacco taxes in WHO Member States

This report includes appendices containing information on the share of total and excise taxes in the price of the most widely sold brand of cigarettes, based on tax policy information collected from each country. This Technical Note contains information on the methodology used by WHO to estimate the share of total and tobacco excise taxes in the price of a pack of 20 cigarettes using country-reported data.

Data collection

Data were collected between July and December 2010 by WHO regional data collectors. The two primary inputs into calculating the share of total and excise taxes were prices and tax rates and structure.

Information collected included the prices of the most widely sold brand of cigarettes, the least-expensive brand and the Marlboro brand for July 2010. Detailed information

was collected in each country on the taxation of cigarettes (and, for some countries in SEAR, bidis) and tobacco tax revenues. Documents such as laws, decrees or other official materials in support of the information provided were also collected.

Data on tax structure were collected through contacts with ministries of finance. The validity of this information was checked against other sources. These sources, including tax law documents, decrees, and official schedules of tax rates and structures and trade information, when available, were either downloaded from ministerial web sites or from other United Nations databases such as Comtrade (http://comtrade.un.org/db/). Other secondary data sources were also purchased for data validation.

The tax data collected focus on indirect taxes levied on tobacco products (e.g. excise taxes of various types, import duties, value added taxes), which usually have the most direct policy

impact on the price of tobacco products. Excise taxes are the most important because they are applied exclusively to tobacco and contribute the most to substantially increasing the price of tobacco products and subsequently reducing consumption. Thus, rates, amounts, functioning and application of excise taxes are central components of the data collected.

Data were not collected on other taxes (e.g., income taxes, corporate taxes) because of the practical difficulty of obtaining information on these taxes and the complexity in estimating their potential impact on price.

The table below describes the types of tax information collected.

Data analysis

Only the price of the most popular brand of cigarettes was considered in the calculation of the tax as a share of the retail price. In the case of countries where different levels of taxes are applied

1. Amount-specific excise taxes	An amount-specific excise tax is a tax *on a selected good* produced for sale within a country, or imported and sold in that country. In general, the tax is collected from the manufacturer/wholesaler or at the point of entry into the country by the importer, in addition to import duties. These taxes come in the form of an amount per pack, per 1000 sticks or per kilogram. Example: US$ 1.50 per pack of 20 cigarettes.
2. Ad valorem excise taxes	An ad valorem excise tax is a tax *on a selected good* produced for sale within a country, or imported and sold in that country. In general, the tax is collected from the manufacturer/wholesaler or at the point of entry into the country by the importer, in addition to import duties. These taxes come in the form of a percentage of the value of a transaction between two independent entities at some point of the production/distribution chain; ad valorem taxes are generally applied to the value of the transactions between the manufacturer and the retailer/wholesaler. Example: 27% of the retail price.
3. Tobacco-specific import duties	An import duty is a tax *on a selected good* imported into a country to be consumed in that country (i.e. the goods are not in transit to another country). In general, the import duties are collected from the importer at the point of entry into the country. These taxes can be either amount-specific or ad valorem. Amount-specific import duties are applied in the same fashion as amount-specific excise taxes. Ad valorem import duties are generally applied to the CIF (cost, insurance, freight) value, i.e. the value of the unloaded consignment that includes the cost of the product itself, insurance, transport and unloading. Example: 50% import duty levied on CIF.
4. Value added taxes	The value added tax (VAT) is a "multi-stage" tax *on all consumer goods and services* applied proportionally to the price the consumer pays for a product. Although manufacturers and wholesalers also participate in the administration and payment of the tax all along the manufacturing/distribution chain, they are all reimbursed through a tax credit system, so that the only person who pays in the end is the final consumer. Most countries that impose a VAT do so on a base that includes any excise tax and customs duty. Example: VAT representing 10% of the retail price.
5. Other taxes	Any other tax that is not called an excise tax, import duty, or VAT but applies to either the quantity of tobacco or to the value of a transaction of tobacco product was reported in the questionnaire, with as much detail as possible regarding what is taxed (base), who pays the tax and how the base is taxed.

on cigarettes based on either length of cigarette, quantity produced or type (e.g. filter vs non-filter), only the rate that applied to the most sold brand was used in the calculation. The only exceptions were made for Canada and the United States where average estimates had to be calculated for prices and taxes because, in addition to federal taxes, different rates were applied by states/provinces, and in some instances by localities.

The import duty was only applied to the most popular brand of cigarettes that were imported into the country. Import duty is not applied on total tax calculation for countries reporting that the most popular brand was produced locally.

"Other taxes" are all other indirect taxes excluding excise, import duties and VAT. These types of taxes were considered excises if they had a special rate applied on tobacco products. For example, Thailand reported the tax earmarked from tobacco and alcohol for the ThaiHealth Promotion Foundation as "other tax". However, since this tax is applied only on tobacco and alcohol products, it acts like an excise tax and it was considered an excise in the calculations.

The next step of the exercise was to convert all tax rates into the same base, in our case, the tax-inclusive retail sales price (hereafter referred to as P). Consider the following example where Country B applies the same ad valorem tax as Country A, but ends up with higher taxation because the tax is applied later in the distribution chain:

Comparing reported ad valorem tax rates without taking into account the stage at which the tax is applied could therefore lead to biased results. This is why WHO used the information provided on tax policy in order to calculate the share of tobacco taxes on the most widely sold pack of cigarettes in the country. This indicator takes into account the exact contribution of all taxes in the price of a cigarette pack and therefore represents the best measure of the magnitude of tobacco taxes.

Calculation

S_{ts} is the share of taxes on the price of a widely consumed brand of cigarettes (20-cigarette pack or equivalent).

$$S_{ts} = S_{as} + S_{av} + S_{id} + S_{VAT} \quad ①$$

Where:

S_{ts} = Total share of taxes on the price of a pack of cigarettes;

S_{as} = Share of amount-specific excise taxes (or equivalent) on the price of a pack of cigarettes;

S_{av} = Share of ad valorem excise taxes (or equivalent) on the price of a pack of cigarettes;

S_{id} = Share of import duties on the price of a pack of cigarettes (if the most popular brand is imported);

S_{VAT} = Share of the value added tax on the price of a pack of cigarettes.

Calculating S_{as} is fairly straightforward and involves dividing the amount for a 20-cigarette pack by the total price. Unlike S_{as}, S_{av} (the share of ad valorem taxes), is much more difficult to calculate and involves making some assumptions. On the other hand, S_{id} is sometimes amount-specific and sometimes value-based. It is therefore calculated the same way as S_{as} if it is amount-specific and the same way as S_{av} if it is value-based. S_{VAT} is usually applied at the end of the taxation process, either on the VAT-exclusive or inclusive retail sales price.

To calculate price, it was assumed that the price of a pack of cigarettes could be expressed as the following: [1]

$$P = [(M + M \times ID) + (M + M \times ID) \times T_{av}\% + T_{as} + \pi] \times (1 + VAT\%) \quad ②$$

Where:

P = Price per pack of 20 cigarettes of the most popular brand consumed locally;

M = Manufacturer's/distributor's price, or import price if the brand is imported;

ID = Total import duties (where applicable) on a pack of 20 cigarettes [2];

T_{av} = Statutory rate of ad valorem tax;

T_{as} = Amount specific excise tax on a pack of 20 cigarettes;

π = Retailer's, wholesaler's and importer's profit margins (sometimes expressed as a mark-up);

VAT = Statutory rate of value added tax.

Changes to this formula were considered based on country-specific conditions such as the existence of ad valorem and specific excise taxes and the tax base, and whether the most popular brand was locally produced or imported. In most cases the base for the ad valorem excise tax was the manufacturer's/distributor's price.

Given knowledge of price (P) and amount-specific excise tax (T_{as}), the shares S_{as} (and, where applicable, S_{id}) are easy to recover. The case of ad valorem taxes (and, where applicable, S_{id}) is more complicated because one needs to recover and separate the base ($M + M \times ID$) of the tax into its component parts in order to calculate the amount

TAX INCLUSIVE RETAIL SALES PRICE OF CIGARETTES	COUNTRY A (US$)	COUNTRY B (US$)
[A] Manufacturer's price (same in both countries)	2.00	2.00
[B] Country A: ad valorem tax on manufacturer's price (20%) = 20% x [A]	**0.40**	-
[C] Countries A and B: specific excise	2.00	2.00
[D] Retailer's and wholesaler's profit margin (same in both countries)	0.20	0.20
[E] Country B: ad valorem tax on retailer's price (20%) = 20% x [A]+[C] +[D]	-	**0.84**
[F] Final price = P = [A]+[B]+[C]+[D]+[E]	4.60	5.04

of ad valorem tax. In most of the cases M was not known (unless specifically reported by the country).

Using equation ②, it is possible to calculate M:

$$M = \frac{\dfrac{P}{1 + VAT\%} - \pi - T_{as}}{(1 + T_{av}\%) \times (1 + ID)} \quad ③$$

Unfortunately, π is unknown and will systematically vary from country to country. For domestically produced most popular brands, we considered π to be nil (i.e. 0) in the calculation of M because the retailer's and wholesaler's margins are assumed to be small. This would result in an overestimation of M and therefore of the base for the ad valorem tax. This will in turn result in an overestimation of the amount of ad valorem tax. Since the goal of this exercise is to measure the share of tobacco taxes in the price of a typical pack of cigarettes, the assumption that the retailer's/wholesaler's profit (π) is nil, therefore, does not penalize countries by underestimating their ad valorem taxes. In light of this, it was decided that unless and until country-specific information was made available to WHO, the retailer's/wholesaler's margin would be assumed to be nil for the domestically produced brands.

However, for those countries where the most popular brand is imported, assuming π to be nil would grossly overestimate the base for the ad valorem tax because the importer's profit needs to be taken into account. The import duty is applied on CIF values, and the consequent excise taxes are applied on import duty inclusive CIF values. The importer's profit or own price is added on tax-inclusive CIF value. For domestically produced cigarettes, the producer's price includes its own profit so it is automatically included in M, but this is not the case for imported products where the tax is imposed on the import duty-inclusive CIF value excluding the importer's profit. So calculating M as in equation ③ would mean assuming the importer's profit to be zero. The importer's profit is assumed to be relatively significant and ignoring it would therefore

overestimate M. For this reason, M had to be estimated differently for imported products: M^* (or the CIF value) was calculated using secondary sources (e.g. data from the United Nations Comtrade database). M^* was normally calculated as the import price of cigarettes in a country (value of imports divided by the quantity of imports for the importing country). However, because of limited data availability and because of inconsistencies in the import data in some cases, the export price was also considered. When both values were available, the higher of the two was selected for the CIF value. Looking more closely at the data, import and export prices sometimes varied greatly depending on the partner considered. In order to take this variation into account, the average import and export prices were weighted for each country by the quantities of the imports/exports coming from the different available partners. When the export price was selected, an additional 10 cents was added to the CIF value because the export price does not include cost, insurance and freight price. The 10 cents value was calculated based on the global difference between import and export prices. The ad valorem and other taxes were then calculated in the same manner as for local cigarettes using M^* as the base, where applicable.

In the case of VAT, in most of the cases the base was P excluding the VAT (or, similarly, the manufacturer's/distributor's price plus all taxes other than VAT). In other words:

$S_{VAT} = VAT\% \times (P - S_{VAT})$, equivalent to
$S_{VAT} = VAT\% \div (1 + VAT\%)$

So in sum the tax rates are calculated this way:

$S_{ts} = S_{id} + S_{as} + S_{av} + S_{VAT}$

$S_{as} = T_{as} \div P$

$S_{av} = (T_{av} \% \times M) \div P$
    or
    $(T_{av} \% \times M^* \times (1 + S_{id})) \div P$
    if the most popular brand was imported

$S_{id} = (T_{ID} \% \times M^*) \div P$
    (if the import duty is value-based)
    or
    $ID \div P$
    (if it is specific)

$S_{VAT} = VAT\% \div (1 + VAT\%)$

Prices

In order to reduce chances of inconsistency in prices collected in 2008 compared to those reported in 2010, the questionnaire distributed among data collectors in 2010 included the brands and prices reported in 2008.[3]

In the case of the most sold brand used for the tax calculation, the information reported in 2010 can be gathered in four groups:

a) brand reported has changed and the price is the same/higher than in 2008;

b) brand reported has changed and the price is lower;

c) brand reported is the same and price is the same/higher;

d) brand reported is the same but price is lower.

The following action was taken for each group:

Groups a and c: no action was taken.

Group a: one concern that could be raised is the comparability of the data when different brands are reported between two years. However, for countries where secondary data were available, the new brand reported often had the same market share as the brand reported in 2008 and they were both in the same price category (22 countries in this group: Albania, Azerbaijan, Bangladesh, Burkina Faso, Cameroon, the Dominican Republic, El Salvador, the Gambia, Ghana, Grenada, Guinea, Honduras, Jordan, Mauritius, Myanmar, Nicaragua, Palau, Panama, the Russian Federation, Saint Kitts and Nevis, Turkey and Zambia).

Groups a and c: another question could be raised here when no tax change was perceived but a higher price was reported in 2010 compared to

2008. It was assumed, however, that the industry tends to increase the price of its product because of inflation, income growth, increase in cost or just to increase its profit margin whenever it has the opportunity to do so.

Groups b and d: an important assumption made was that prices could not have gone down from 2008 to 2010 unless there was a tax decrease (e.g. Myanmar). Because of positive inflation and increase in incomes the price cannot go down. Therefore, the prices had to be revised:

- In group b: the brand and price for 2008 were replaced by the data reported in 2010, resulting in no change between the two years. The 2010 price was chosen as a reference because in many regions the data collection process was improved, involving data collectors more knowledgeable in tobacco tax and price issues (12 countries in this group: Antigua and Barbuda, the Bahamas, the Comoros, Cook Islands, Ecuador, Iran (Islamic Republic of), the Philippines, Saint Lucia, Sierra Leone, Swaziland, Tonga and Tuvalu).

- In group d: it seemed odd to experience a reduction in the price of a same brand between 2008 and 2010 while no tax changes or other major events occurred. It was therefore assumed that a mistake was made in the reporting, so the price for 2008 was also replaced by the price reported in 2010, resulting in no change in the price between the two years (four countries in this group: Afghanistan, Dominica, Maldives and Micronesia (Federated States of)).

Considerations in interpreting tax share changes

It is important to note that the change in the tax as a share of the price is not only dependent on tax changes but also on changes in the price. Therefore, despite an increase in the tax, the tax share might remain the same or go down.

Similarly, a tax share might increase despite no change or a decrease in the tax.

In the current database, there are cases of tax increases between 2008 and 2010 where the share of tax as a percentage of price either did not change or went down. This is mainly due to the fact that, in absolute terms, the increase in the price is larger than the increase in the tax (particularly in the case of specific excise tax increases).

For example, in Uzbekistan, the excise tax increased from 104.1 sums per pack in 2008 to 143.2 sums per pack in 2010 (a non-negligible increase) while the price of the most sold brand increased from 700 to 1100 sums per pack. In terms of tax share, however, the excise represented 14.87% (104.1/700) of the price in 2008 while it represented 13.02% (143.2/1100) of the price in 2010. This is because the prices increased to a larger extent than taxes did.

Conversely, there are also cases where increases (decreases) in the tax as a share of the price occurred despite no change in the tax. In the current database, this was due to one of the following reasons:

- Price increased independently of tax change (leading to a decrease in the tax share).

- In the case of imported products, the CIF value had to be estimated using secondary data, as explained above. The CIF values are provided in US$, so they were converted into the local currency. This exercise introduced other external factors that had also an impact on the results for taxes as a percentage of the retail price (one of the following reasons or a combination of the two):

  – CIF value in US$ decreased (increased) between 2008 and 2010, making the base for the application of the tax lower (higher), therefore leading to a lower (higher) tax percentage despite no change in the tax rate.

  – The exchange rate decreased (increased)

between 2008 and 2010, leading to a lower (higher) CIF value in the local currency, leading also to a lower (higher) base for the application of the tax and also leading to a lower (higher) tax percentage.

1   This formula applies when the ad valorem tax is applied on the manufacturer's/distributor's price, the import duty is applied on the manufacturer's/distributor's price or the CIF value, and the VAT is applied on the VAT-exclusive retail price. Other scenarios exist (e.g. Ad valorem rate applies to the retail price) but they are not described here because they are usually more straightforward to calculate.

2   Import duties may vary depending on the country of origin in cases of preferential trade agreements. WHO tried to determine the origin of the pack and relevance of using such rates where possible.

3   The brands are used for internal purposes for data validation and are not published in this report.

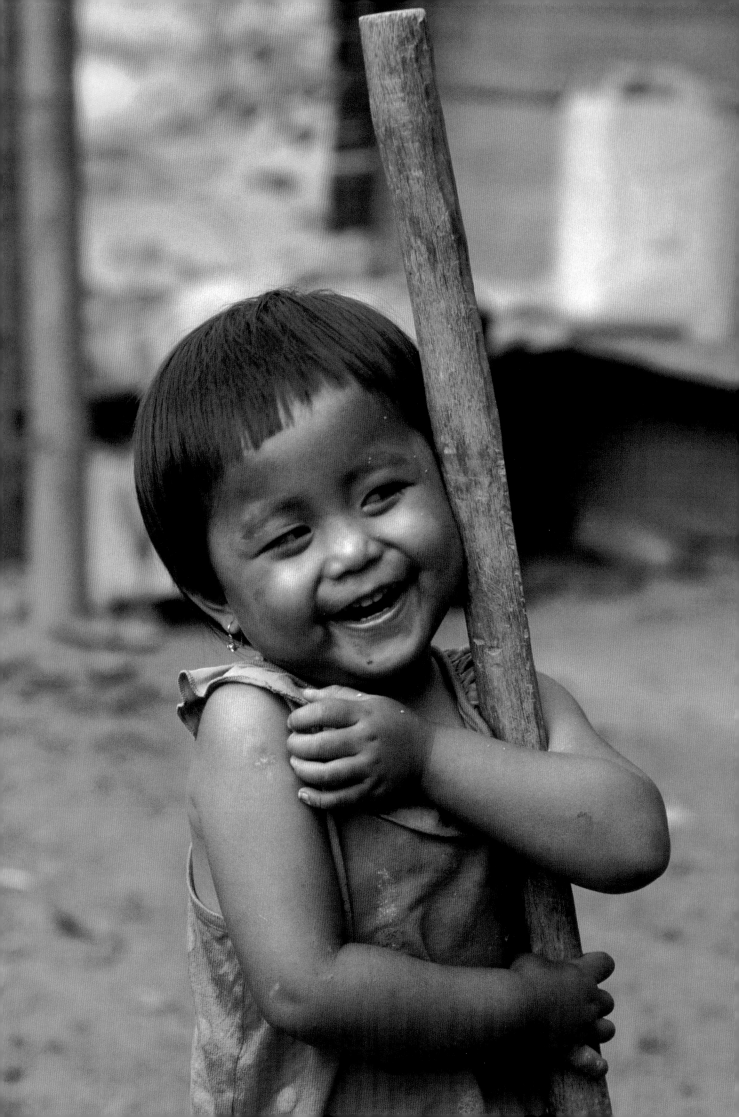

APPENDIX I: **REGIONAL SUMMARY OF MPOWER MEASURES**

Appendix I provides an overview of selected tobacco control policies. For each WHO region an overview table is presented that includes information on monitoring and prevalence, smoke-free environments, treatment of tobacco dependence, health warnings and packaging, advertising, promotion and sponsorship bans, and taxation levels, based on the methodology outlined in Technical Note I.

Country-level data were often but not always provided with supporting documents such as laws, regulations, policy documents, etc. Available documents were reviewed by WHO and answers were amended accordingly, especially for Member States that reported meeting the highest standards.

This review, however, does not constitute a thorough and complete legal analysis of each country's legislation. Except for smoke-free environments, data were collected at the national/federal level only and, therefore, provide incomplete policy coverage for Member States where subnational governments play an active role in tobacco control.

Age-standardized prevalence estimates for both sexes combined were produced by applying global population weights for males and females to the age-standardized adult male and female daily smoking prevalence rates (as presented in Appendix VII). Global male and female population weights were obtained from the United Nations population data for 2010.

Africa

Table 1.0.1
Summary of MPOWER measures

... Data not reported/not available.

− Data not required/not applicable.

COUNTRY	AGE- AND SEX-STANDARDIZED ADULT DAILY SMOKING PREVALENCE (2009)	M MONITORING	P SMOKE-FREE POLICIES (LINES REPRESENT LEVEL OF COMPLIANCE)	O CESSATION PROGRAMMES	W WARNINGS — WARNING LABELS	W WARNINGS — MASS MEDIA	E ADVERTISING BANS (LINES REPRESENT LEVEL OF COMPLIANCE)	R TAXATION
Algeria	...							55%
Angola	...		...					...
Benin	6%							43%
Botswana	...						...	48%
Burkina Faso	12%		−					23%
Burundi	...							56%
Cameroon	6%							26%
Cape Verde	6%							26%
Central African Republic	...							29%
Chad	11%							33%
Comoros	14%							70%
Congo	4%		»					32%
Côte d'Ivoire	9%							34%
Democratic Republic of the Congo	5%							25%
Equatorial Guinea	...		...»					...
Eritrea	5%							55%
Ethiopia	3%						...»	55%
Gabon	9%							22%
Gambia	15%							66%
Ghana	5%						»	27%
Guinea	12%							43%
Guinea-Bissau	...				»			44%
Kenya	10%							64%
Lesotho	...		...				...»	41%
Liberia	...							46%
Madagascar	...							76%
Malawi	11%							...
Mali	14%							22%
Mauritania	15%		||»					20%
Mauritius	13%							72%
Mozambique	7%							60%
Namibia	15%		...				...	46%
Niger	3%							27%
Nigeria	5%							21%
Rwanda	...							66%
Sao Tome and Principe	4%							11%
Senegal	7%							42%
Seychelles	11%							68%
Sierra Leone	22%							39%
South Africa	13%							53%
Swaziland	6%							53%
Togo	...							32%
Uganda	7%		|||||☆					45%
United Republic of Tanzania	10%						...	26%
Zambia	11%							45%
Zimbabwe	14%							52%

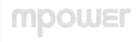

CHANGE SINCE 2008

P SMOKE-FREE POLICIES	O CESSATION PROGRAMMES	W WARNING LABELS	E ADVERTISING BANS	R TAXATION

CHANGE IN POWER INDICATOR GROUP, UP OR DOWN, SINCE 2008

ADULT DAILY SMOKING PREVALENCE*: AGE- AND SEX-STANDARDIZED PREVALENCE RATES FOR ADULT DAILY SMOKERS OF TOBACCO (BOTH SEXES COMBINED), 2009

. . .	Estimates not available
	30% or more
	From 20% to 29%
	From 15% to 19%
	Less than 15%

* The figures should be used strictly for the purpose of drawing comparisons across countries and must not be used to estimate absolute number of daily tobacco smokers in a country.

MONITORING: PREVALENCE DATA

	No known data or no recent data or data that are not both recent and representative
	Recent and representative data for either adults or youth
	Recent and representative data for both adults and youth
	Recent, representative and periodic data for both adults and youth

SMOKE-FREE POLICIES:
POLICIES ON SMOKE-FREE ENVIRONMENTS

	Data not reported
	Up to two public places completely smoke-free
	Three to five public places completely smoke-free
	Six to seven public places completely smoke-free
	All public places completely smoke-free (or at least 90% of the population covered by complete subnational smoke-free legislation)

CESSATION PROGRAMMES:
TREATMENT OF TOBACCO DEPENDENCE

	Data not reported
	None
	NRT and/or some cessation services (neither cost-covered)
	NRT and/or some cessation services (at least one of which is cost-covered)
	National quit line, and both NRT and some cessation services cost-covered

WARNINGS:
HEALTH WARNINGS ON CIGARETTE PACKAGES

	Data not reported
	No warnings or small warnings
	Medium size warnings missing some appropriate characteristics OR large warnings missing many appropriate characteristics
	Medium size warnings with all appropriate characteristics OR large warnings missing some appropriate characteristics
	Large warnings with all appropriate characteristics

WARNINGS:
ANTI-TOBACCO MASS MEDIA CAMPAIGNS

	Data not reported
	No campaign conducted between January 2009 and August 2010 with duration of at least three weeks
	Campaign conducted with 1–4 appropriate characteristics
	Campaign conducted with 5–6 appropriate characteristics
	Campaign conducted with all appropriate characteristics

ADVERTISING BANS:
BANS ON ADVERTISING, PROMOTION AND SPONSORSHIP

	Data not reported
	Complete absence of ban, or ban that does not cover national television, radio and print media
	Ban on national television, radio and print media only
	Ban on national television, radio and print media as well as on some but not all other forms of direct and/or indirect advertising
	Ban on all forms of direct and indirect advertising

TAXATION: SHARE OF TOTAL TAXES IN THE RETAIL PRICE OF THE MOST WIDELY SOLD BRAND OF CIGARETTES

	Data not reported
	≤ 25% of retail price is tax
	26–50% of retail price is tax
	51–75% of retail price is tax
	>75% of retail price is tax

COMPLIANCE: COMPLIANCE WITH BANS ON ADVERTISING, PROMOTION AND SPONSORSHIP, AND ADHERENCE TO SMOKE-FREE POLICY

‖‖‖‖‖‖‖‖ ‖‖‖‖‖‖‖‖ ‖‖‖‖‖‖‖‖	Complete compliance (8/10 to 10/10)
‖‖‖‖‖‖‖ ‖‖‖‖‖‖ ‖‖‖‖‖ ‖‖‖‖ ‖‖‖	Moderate compliance (3/10 to 7/10)
‖ |	Minimal compliance (0/10 to 2/10)

SYMBOLS LEGEND

☆	Separate, completely enclosed smoking rooms are allowed under very strict conditions (refer to Technical Note I for more details)
⊙	Policy adopted but not implemented by 31 December 2010
»	Data not substantiated by a copy of the legislation
▲ ▼	Change in POWER indicator group, up or down, between 2008 and 2010. Some 2008 data were revised in 2010. 2010 grouping rules were applied to both years

Refer to Technical Note I
for definitions of categories

The Americas

Table 1.0.2
Summary of MPOWER measures

. . . Data not reported/not available.

2010 INDICATOR AND COMPLIANCE

COUNTRY	AGE- AND SEX-STANDARDIZED ADULT DAILY SMOKING PREVALENCE (2009)	M MONITORING	P SMOKE-FREE POLICIES (LINES REPRESENT LEVEL OF COMPLIANCE)	O CESSATION PROGRAMMES	W WARNINGS — WARNING LABELS	W WARNINGS — MASS MEDIA	E ADVERTISING BANS (LINES REPRESENT LEVEL OF COMPLIANCE)	R TAXATION
Antigua and Barbuda	. . .		. . .					12%
Argentina	22%							76%
Bahamas	. . .							31%
Barbados	5%							48%
Belize	4%							21%
Bolivia (Plurinational State of)	6%		|||||				|||||	42%
Brazil	15%		|||||				||||||	60%
Canada	14%		||||||||				|||||||||	67%
Chile	34%		|||||				|||||	76%
Colombia	. . .		|||||				|||||	50%
Costa Rica	6%		|||||					56%
Cuba	. . .							. . .
Dominica	5%							26%
Dominican Republic	13%		|||||					57%
Ecuador	. . .		|||||					64%
El Salvador	. . .								55%
Grenada	. . .							49%
Guatemala	4%		|||||				||	57%
Guyana	9%		||					21%
Haiti	. . .							. . .
Honduras	. . .		⊙		⊙		⊙	39%
Jamaica	. . .						||||||	51%
Mexico	8%		|||| ☆				||||||	63%
Nicaragua	. . .		. . . ⊙		⊙		. . . ⊙	29%
Panama	. . .		||||||||				||||||||	47%
Paraguay	15%		||||||||					18%
Peru	. . .						|||	50%
Saint Kitts and Nevis	5%							14%
Saint Lucia	19%							31%
Saint Vincent and the Grenadines	11%							16%
Suriname	. . .							50%
Trinidad and Tobago	18%		|||||				|||||	34%
United States of America	16%				⊙		||||||	45%
Uruguay	22%		||||||||				|||||||||	72%
Venezuela (Bolivarian Republic of)	. . .		||||||||				||||||	71%

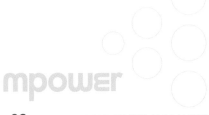

CHANGE SINCE 2008

P SMOKE-FREE POLICIES	O CESSATION PROGRAMMES	W WARNING LABELS	E ADVERTISING BANS	R TAXATION
CHANGE IN POWER INDICATOR GROUP, UP OR DOWN, SINCE 2008					
				▲
▲				
▼				
			▲	
		▲	▲	
				▲
				▼
▲		▲	▲	
				▲
	▲			
▲		▲		▲
▲		▲		
				▼
▲				
		▲		

ADULT DAILY SMOKING PREVALENCE*: AGE- AND SEX-STANDARDIZED PREVALENCE RATES FOR ADULT DAILY SMOKERS OF TOBACCO (BOTH SEXES COMBINED), 2009

. . .	Estimates not available
	30% or more
	From 20% to 29%
	From 15% to 19%
	Less than 15%

* The figures should be used strictly for the purpose of drawing comparisons across countries and must not be used to estimate absolute number of daily tobacco smokers in a country.

MONITORING: PREVALENCE DATA

	No known data or no recent data or data that are not both recent and representative
	Recent and representative data for either adults or youth
	Recent and representative data for both adults and youth
	Recent, representative and periodic data for both adults and youth

SMOKE-FREE POLICIES: POLICIES ON SMOKE-FREE ENVIRONMENTS

	Data not reported
	Up to two public places completely smoke-free
	Three to five public places completely smoke-free
	Six to seven public places completely smoke-free
	All public places completely smoke-free (or at least 90% of the population covered by complete subnational smoke-free legislation)

CESSATION PROGRAMMES: TREATMENT OF TOBACCO DEPENDENCE

	Data not reported
	None
	NRT and/or some cessation services (neither cost-covered)
	NRT and/or some cessation services (at least one of which is cost-covered)
	National quit line, and both NRT and some cessation services cost-covered

WARNINGS: HEALTH WARNINGS ON CIGARETTE PACKAGES

	Data not reported
	No warnings or small warnings
	Medium size warnings missing some appropriate characteristics OR large warnings missing many appropriate characteristics
	Medium size warnings with all appropriate characteristics OR large warnings missing some appropriate characteristics
	Large warnings with all appropriate characteristics

WARNINGS: ANTI-TOBACCO MASS MEDIA CAMPAIGNS

	Data not reported
	No campaign conducted between January 2009 and August 2010 with duration of at least three weeks
	Campaign conducted with 1–4 appropriate characteristics
	Campaign conducted with 5–6 appropriate characteristics
	Campaign conducted with all appropriate characteristics

ADVERTISING BANS: BANS ON ADVERTISING, PROMOTION AND SPONSORSHIP

	Data not reported
	Complete absence of ban, or ban that does not cover national television, radio and print media
	Ban on national television, radio and print media only
	Ban on national television, radio and print media as well as on some but not all other forms of direct and/or indirect advertising
	Ban on all forms of direct and indirect advertising

TAXATION: SHARE OF TOTAL TAXES IN THE RETAIL PRICE OF THE MOST WIDELY SOLD BRAND OF CIGARETTES

	Data not reported
	≤ 25% of retail price is tax
	26–50% of retail price is tax
	51–75% of retail price is tax
	>75% of retail price is tax

COMPLIANCE: COMPLIANCE WITH BANS ON ADVERTISING, PROMOTION AND SPONSORSHIP, AND ADHERENCE TO SMOKE-FREE POLICY

‖‖‖‖‖‖	Complete compliance (8/10 to 10/10)
‖‖‖‖‖	Moderate compliance (3/10 to 7/10)
‖	Minimal compliance (0/10 to 2/10)

SYMBOLS LEGEND

☆	Separate, completely enclosed smoking rooms are allowed under very strict conditions (refer to Technical Note I for more details)
⊙	Policy adopted but not implemented by 31 December 2010
▲▼	Change in POWER indicator group, up or down, between 2008 and 2010. Some 2008 data were revised in 2010. 2010 grouping rules were applied to both years

Refer to Technical Note I
for definitions of categories

South-East Asia

Table 1.0.3
Summary of MPOWER measures

. . . Data not reported/not available.

2010 INDICATOR AND COMPLIANCE

COUNTRY	AGE- AND SEX-STANDARDIZED ADULT DAILY SMOKING PREVALENCE (2009)	M MONITORING	P SMOKE-FREE POLICIES (LINES REPRESENT LEVEL OF COMPLIANCE)	O CESSATION PROGRAMMES	W WARNINGS — WARNING LABELS	W WARNINGS — MASS MEDIA	E ADVERTISING BANS (LINES REPRESENT LEVEL OF COMPLIANCE)	R TAXATION
Bangladesh	22%		‖‖				‖‖‖‖‖‖	68%
Bhutan	. . .		‖‖‖‖				‖‖‖‖‖‖‖‖	. . .
Democratic People's Republic of Korea	. . .		. . .					. . .
India	12%		‖‖‖‖				‖‖‖‖‖	46%
Indonesia	29%		‖					54%
Maldives	24%		. . . ⊙		⊙		‖‖‖‖‖‖‖ ⊙	32%
Myanmar	18%		‖‖				‖‖‖‖‖	50%
Nepal	28%		‖‖‖‖				‖‖‖‖	29%
Sri Lanka	11%		‖‖‖‖				‖‖‖‖‖	73%
Thailand	20%		‖‖‖‖‖‖				‖‖‖‖‖‖	69%
Timor-Leste	. . .		‖‖‖‖ »					. . .

mpower

CHANGE SINCE 2008

P SMOKE-FREE POLICIES	O CESSATION PROGRAMMES	W WARNING LABELS	E ADVERTISING BANS	R TAXATION
CHANGE IN POWER INDICATOR GROUP, UP OR DOWN, SINCE 2008				
			▲	
▲				
▲				
				▼
▲			▲	▲
▲				
	▲			

ADULT DAILY SMOKING PREVALENCE*: AGE- AND SEX-STANDARDIZED PREVALENCE RATES FOR ADULT DAILY SMOKERS OF TOBACCO (BOTH SEXES COMBINED), 2009

...	Estimates not available
	30% or more
	From 20% to 29%
	From 15% to 19%
	Less than 15%

* The figures should be used strictly for the purpose of drawing comparisons across countries and must not be used to estimate absolute number of daily tobacco smokers in a country.

MONITORING: PREVALENCE DATA

	No known data or no recent data or data that are not both recent and representative
	Recent and representative data for either adults or youth
	Recent and representative data for both adults and youth
	Recent, representative and periodic data for both adults and youth

SMOKE-FREE POLICIES:
POLICIES ON SMOKE-FREE ENVIRONMENTS

	Data not reported
	Up to two public places completely smoke-free
	Three to five public places completely smoke-free
	Six to seven public places completely smoke-free
	All public places completely smoke-free (or at least 90% of the population covered by complete subnational smoke-free legislation)

CESSATION PROGRAMMES:
TREATMENT OF TOBACCO DEPENDENCE

	Data not reported
	None
	NRT and/or some cessation services (neither cost-covered)
	NRT and/or some cessation services (at least one of which is cost-covered)
	National quit line, and both NRT and some cessation services cost-covered

WARNINGS:
HEALTH WARNINGS ON CIGARETTE PACKAGES

	Data not reported
	No warnings or small warnings
	Medium size warnings missing some appropriate characteristics OR large warnings missing many appropriate characteristics
	Medium size warnings with all appropriate characteristics OR large warnings missing some appropriate characteristics
	Large warnings with all appropriate characteristics

WARNINGS:
ANTI-TOBACCO MASS MEDIA CAMPAIGNS

	Data not reported
	No campaign conducted between January 2009 and August 2010 with duration of at least three weeks
	Campaign conducted with 1–4 appropriate characteristics
	Campaign conducted with 5–6 appropriate characteristics
	Campaign conducted with all appropriate characteristics

ADVERTISING BANS:
BANS ON ADVERTISING, PROMOTION AND SPONSORSHIP

	Data not reported
	Complete absence of ban, or ban that does not cover national television, radio and print media
	Ban on national television, radio and print media only
	Ban on national television, radio and print media as well as on some but not all other forms of direct and/or indirect advertising
	Ban on all forms of direct and indirect advertising

TAXATION: SHARE OF TOTAL TAXES IN THE RETAIL PRICE OF THE MOST WIDELY SOLD BRAND OF CIGARETTES

	Data not reported
	≤ 25% of retail price is tax
	26–50% of retail price is tax
	51–75% of retail price is tax
	>75% of retail price is tax

COMPLIANCE: COMPLIANCE WITH BANS ON ADVERTISING, PROMOTION AND SPONSORSHIP, AND ADHERENCE TO SMOKE-FREE POLICY

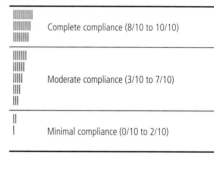

Complete compliance (8/10 to 10/10)

Moderate compliance (3/10 to 7/10)

Minimal compliance (0/10 to 2/10)

SYMBOLS LEGEND

⊙	Policy adopted but not implemented by 31 December 2010
»	Data not substantiated by a copy of the legislation
▲ ▼	Change in POWER indicator group, up or down, between 2008 and 2010. Some 2008 data were revised in 2010. 2010 grouping rules were applied to both years

Refer to Technical Note I
for definitions of categories

Europe

Table 1.0.4
Summary of MPOWER measures

... Data not reported/not available.

– Data not required/not applicable.

COUNTRY	AGE- AND SEX-STANDARDIZED ADULT DAILY SMOKING PREVALENCE (2009)	M MONITORING	P SMOKE-FREE POLICIES (LINES REPRESENT LEVEL OF COMPLIANCE)	O CESSATION PROGRAMMES	W WARNINGS (WARNING LABELS)	W WARNINGS (MASS MEDIA)	E ADVERTISING BANS (LINES REPRESENT LEVEL OF COMPLIANCE)	R TAXATION
Albania	36%							53%
Andorra	31%							58%
Armenia	23%							24%
Austria	44%							73%
Azerbaijan	...							26%
Belarus	25%							27%
Belgium	21%		— ☆					76%
Bosnia and Herzegovina	37%							70%
Bulgaria	32%							89%
Croatia	29%							72%
Cyprus	...							72%
Czech Republic	27%							79%
Denmark	21%							75%
Estonia	27%						...	83%
Finland	17%							79%
France	27%		... ☆				...	80%
Georgia	27%		...					61%
Germany	25%							74%
Greece	49%							86%
Hungary	32%							79%
Iceland	17%							56%
Ireland	...							79%
Israel	...						...	82%
Italy	22%		— ☆					75%
Kazakhstan	20%							27%
Kyrgyzstan	20%							18%
Latvia	29%							81%
Lithuania	28%							77%
Luxembourg	...		...				...	70%
Malta	22%				⊙			76%
Monaco	...							...
Montenegro	...							65%
Netherlands	22%							73%
Norway	20%				⊙			72%
Poland	27%							86%
Portugal	20%		...					79%
Republic of Moldova	20%							30%
Romania	29%							83%
Russian Federation	36%							35%
San Marino	...							74%
Serbia	29%							72%
Slovakia	23%							83%
Slovenia	22%							76%
Spain	28%		⊙					78%
Sweden	...							72%
Switzerland	19%							63%
Tajikistan	...							22%
The former Yugoslav Republic of Macedonia	...							72%
Turkey	27%							78%
Turkmenistan	...							49%
Ukraine	28%				⊙			70%
United Kingdom of Great Britain and Northern Ireland	16%							77%
Uzbekistan	10%							30%

CHANGE SINCE 2008

P SMOKE-FREE POLICIES	O CESSATION PROGRAMMES	W WARNING LABELS	E ADVERTISING BANS	R TAXATION
CHANGE IN POWER INDICATOR GROUP, UP OR DOWN, SINCE 2008				
				▲
				▲
▼				
▲				
		▲		
			▲	▼
▲				▲
	▲			▲
				▲
				▲
				▲
			▲	▼
▲	▲			▲
				▲
▲		▲		
				▲
	▲			
		▲		
				▲
				▲
	▲			
▲				
				▲
▲		▲		
	▲	▲		▲
▲		▲		▲
	▲			

ADULT DAILY SMOKING PREVALENCE*: AGE- AND SEX-STANDARDIZED PREVALENCE RATES FOR ADULT DAILY SMOKERS OF TOBACCO (BOTH SEXES COMBINED), 2009

. . .	Estimates not available
	30% or more
	From 20% to 29%
	From 15% to 19%
	Less than 15%

* The figures should be used strictly for the purpose of drawing comparisons across countries and must not be used to estimate absolute number of daily tobacco smokers in a country.

MONITORING: PREVALENCE DATA

	No known data or no recent data or data that are not both recent and representative
	Recent and representative data for either adults or youth
	Recent and representative data for both adults and youth
	Recent, representative and periodic data for both adults and youth

SMOKE-FREE POLICIES: POLICIES ON SMOKE-FREE ENVIRONMENTS

	Data not reported
	Up to two public places completely smoke-free
	Three to five public places completely smoke-free
	Six to seven public places completely smoke-free
	All public places completely smoke-free (or at least 90% of the population covered by complete subnational smoke-free legislation)

CESSATION PROGRAMMES: TREATMENT OF TOBACCO DEPENDENCE

	Data not reported
	None
	NRT and/or some cessation services (neither cost-covered)
	NRT and/or some cessation services (at least one of which is cost-covered)
	National quit line, and both NRT and some cessation services cost covered

WARNINGS: HEALTH WARNINGS ON CIGARETTE PACKAGES

	Data not reported
	No warnings or small warnings
	Medium size warnings missing some appropriate characteristics OR large warnings missing many appropriate characteristics
	Medium size warnings with all appropriate characteristics OR large warnings missing some appropriate characteristics
	Large warnings with all appropriate characteristics

WARNINGS: ANTI-TOBACCO MASS MEDIA CAMPAIGNS

	Data not reported
	No campaign conducted between January 2009 and August 2010 with duration of at least three weeks
	Campaign conducted with 1–4 appropriate characteristics
	Campaign conducted with 5–6 appropriate characteristics
	Campaign conducted with all appropriate characteristics

ADVERTISING BANS: BANS ON ADVERTISING, PROMOTION AND SPONSORSHIP

	Data not reported
	Complete absence of ban, or ban that does not cover national television, radio and print media
	Ban on national television, radio and print media only
	Ban on national television, radio and print media as well as on some but not all other forms of direct and/or indirect advertising
	Ban on all forms of direct and indirect advertising

TAXATION: SHARE OF TOTAL TAXES IN THE RETAIL PRICE OF THE MOST WIDELY SOLD BRAND OF CIGARETTES

	Data not reported
	$\leq$ 25% of retail price is tax
	26–50% of retail price is tax
	51–75% of retail price is tax
	>75% of retail price is tax

COMPLIANCE: COMPLIANCE WITH BANS ON ADVERTISING, PROMOTION AND SPONSORSHIP, AND ADHERENCE TO SMOKE-FREE POLICY

‖‖‖‖‖‖‖‖	Complete compliance (8/10 to 10/10)
‖‖‖‖‖	Moderate compliance (3/10 to 7/10)
‖	Minimal compliance (0/10 to 2/10)

SYMBOLS LEGEND

✿	Separate, completely enclosed smoking rooms are allowed under very strict conditions (refer to Technical Note I for more details)
⊙	Policy adopted but not implemented by 31 December 2010
▲ ▼	Change in POWER indicator group, up or down, between 2008 and 2010. Some 2008 data were revised in 2010. 2010 grouping rules were applied to both years

Refer to Technical Note I
for definitions of categories

Eastern Mediterranean

Table 1.0.5
Summary of MPOWER measures

... Data not reported/not available.
< Refers to a territory.

2010 INDICATOR AND COMPLIANCE

COUNTRY	AGE- AND SEX-STANDARDIZED ADULT DAILY SMOKING PREVALENCE (2009)	M MONITORING	P SMOKE-FREE POLICIES (LINES REPRESENT LEVEL OF COMPLIANCE)	O CESSATION PROGRAMMES	W WARNINGS — WARNING LABELS	W WARNINGS — MASS MEDIA	E ADVERTISING BANS (LINES REPRESENT LEVEL OF COMPLIANCE)	R TAXATION
Afghanistan	...		...				...	9%
Bahrain	19%						|||||||	29%
Djibouti	...		...				...	31%
Egypt	19%		||				|||||||	74%
Iran (Islamic Republic of)	11%		|||||||				|||||||	13%
Iraq	15%						||||	23%
Jordan	26%		||||||				||||	75%
Kuwait	17%						||||	34%
Lebanon	37%		||					47%
Libyan Arab Jamahiriya	23%		|||				|||||||	2%
Morocco	16%		...				...	...
Oman	4%						|||||||	31%
Pakistan	17%								|||||||	62%
Qatar	...						|||||||	33%
Saudi Arabia	9%		...				... »	29%
Somalia	...		|||| »					10%
Sudan	12%						|||	72%
Syrian Arab Republic	...		|||||				|||||||	33%
Tunisia	31%						|||||||	65%
United Arab Emirates	7%		|||||||				||||||	29%
West Bank and Gaza Strip <	...		||||||||				|||||||	78%
Yemen	21%						|||||	53%

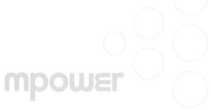

CHANGE SINCE 2008

P SMOKE-FREE POLICIES	O CESSATION PROGRAMMES	W WARNING LABELS	E ADVERTISING BANS	R TAXATION
CHANGE IN POWER INDICATOR GROUP, UP OR DOWN, SINCE 2008				
			▲	
				▼
▲				
▲		▲		
▲			▲	

ADULT DAILY SMOKING PREVALENCE*: AGE- AND SEX-STANDARDIZED PREVALENCE RATES FOR ADULT DAILY SMOKERS OF TOBACCO (BOTH SEXES COMBINED), 2009

. . .	Estimates not available
	30% or more
	From 20% to 29%
	From 15% to 19%
	Less than 15%

* The figures should be used strictly for the purpose of drawing comparisons across countries and must not be used to estimate absolute number of daily tobacco smokers in a country.

MONITORING: PREVALENCE DATA

	No known data or no recent data or data that are not both recent and representative
	Recent and representative data for either adults or youth
	Recent and representative data for both adults and youth
	Recent, representative and periodic data for both adults and youth

SMOKE-FREE POLICIES: POLICIES ON SMOKE-FREE ENVIRONMENTS

	Data not reported
	Up to two public places completely smoke-free
	Three to five public places completely smoke-free
	Six to seven public places completely smoke-free
	All public places completely smoke-free (or at least 90% of the population covered by complete subnational smoke-free legislation)

CESSATION PROGRAMMES: TREATMENT OF TOBACCO DEPENDENCE

	Data not reported
	None
	NRT and/or some cessation services (neither cost-covered)
	NRT and/or some cessation services (at least one of which is cost-covered)
	National quit line, and both NRT and some cessation services cost-covered

WARNINGS: HEALTH WARNINGS ON CIGARETTE PACKAGES

	Data not reported
	No warnings or small warnings
	Medium size warnings missing some appropriate characteristics OR large warnings missing many appropriate characteristics
	Medium size warnings with all appropriate characteristics OR large warnings missing some appropriate characteristics
	Large warnings with all appropriate characteristics

WARNINGS: ANTI-TOBACCO MASS MEDIA CAMPAIGNS

	Data not reported
	No campaign conducted between January 2009 and August 2010 with duration of at least three weeks
	Campaign conducted with 1–4 appropriate characteristics
	Campaign conducted with 5–6 appropriate characteristics
	Campaign conducted with all appropriate characteristics

ADVERTISING BANS: BANS ON ADVERTISING, PROMOTION AND SPONSORSHIP

	Data not reported
	Complete absence of ban, or ban that does not cover national television, radio and print media
	Ban on national television, radio and print media only
	Ban on national television, radio and print media as well as on some but not all other forms of direct and/or indirect advertising
	Ban on all forms of direct and indirect advertising

TAXATION: SHARE OF TOTAL TAXES IN THE RETAIL PRICE OF THE MOST WIDELY SOLD BRAND OF CIGARETTES

	Data not reported
	≤ 25% of retail price is tax
	26–50% of retail price is tax
	51–75% of retail price is tax
	>75% of retail price is tax

COMPLIANCE: COMPLIANCE WITH BANS ON ADVERTISING, PROMOTION AND SPONSORSHIP, AND ADHERENCE TO SMOKE-FREE POLICY

‖‖‖‖‖‖	Complete compliance (8/10 to 10/10)
‖‖‖‖	Moderate compliance (3/10 to 7/10)
‖	Minimal compliance (0/10 to 2/10)

SYMBOLS LEGEND

»	Data not substantiated by a copy of the legislation
⊙	Policy adopted but not implemented by 31 December 2010
▲ ▼	Change in POWER indicator group, up or down, between 2008 and 2010. Some 2008 data were revised in 2010. 2010 grouping rules were applied to both years

Refer to Technical Note I
for definitions of categories

Western Pacific

Table 1.0.6
Summary of MPOWER measures

... Data not reported/not available.

— Data not required/not applicable.

COUNTRY	AGE- AND SEX-STANDARDIZED ADULT DAILY SMOKING PREVALENCE (2009)	M MONITORING	P SMOKE-FREE POLICIES (LINES REPRESENT LEVEL OF COMPLIANCE)	O CESSATION PROGRAMMES	W WARNINGS — WARNING LABELS	W WARNINGS — MASS MEDIA	E ADVERTISING BANS (LINES REPRESENT LEVEL OF COMPLIANCE)	R TAXATION
Australia	17%		—				‖‖‖‖‖	64%
Brunei Darussalam	13%		‖‖‖				‖‖‖‖‖	63%
Cambodia	22%							20%
China	23%		‖				‖‖	41%
Cook Islands	33%		‖‖‖				‖‖‖‖‖	78%
Fiji	8%		...				‖‖‖‖‖	...
Japan	25%							63%
Kiribati	55%							50%
Lao People's Democratic Republic	23%		...				... »	39%
Malaysia	21%						‖‖‖‖‖	52%
Marshall Islands	17%		...				...	36%
Micronesia (Federated States of)	19%		»					72%
Mongolia	24%		‖‖				‖‖‖	33%
Nauru	47%		... ⊙				... ⊙	42%
New Zealand	20%		‖‖‖‖				‖‖‖‖‖	72%
Niue	...							63%
Palau	19%		‖‖‖‖‖					57%
Papua New Guinea	41%						‖‖‖	...
Philippines	23%		‖‖‖				‖‖‖	63%
Republic of Korea	25%		‖‖‖‖				‖‖‖‖	62%
Samoa	...		‖‖‖				‖‖‖‖‖	61%
Singapore	15%		‖‖‖‖‖				‖‖‖‖‖	67%
Solomon Islands	27%		... ⊙		⊙		... ⊙	...
Tonga	23%		...				...	68%
Tuvalu	31%		‖‖‖				‖‖‖‖‖	19%
Vanuatu	11%						...	60%
Viet Nam	20%		‖‖ »				‖‖‖ »	42%

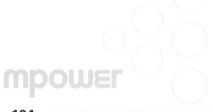

CHANGE SINCE 2008

P SMOKE-FREE POLICIES	O CESSATION PROGRAMMES	W WARNING LABELS	E ADVERTISING BANS	R TAXATION
CHANGE IN POWER INDICATOR GROUP, UP OR DOWN, SINCE 2008				
		▲		
				▲
▲			▲	
				▼
		▲		
▲		▲	▲	

ADULT DAILY SMOKING PREVALENCE*: AGE- AND SEX-STANDARDIZED PREVALENCE RATES FOR ADULT DAILY SMOKERS OF TOBACCO (BOTH SEXES COMBINED), 2009

. . .	Estimates not available
	30% or more
	From 20% to 29%
	From 15% to 19%
	Less than 15%

* The figures should be used strictly for the purpose of drawing comparisons across countries and must not be used to estimate absolute number of daily tobacco smokers in a country.

MONITORING: PREVALENCE DATA

	No known data or no recent data or data that are not both recent and representative
	Recent and representative data for either adults or youth
	Recent and representative data for both adults and youth
	Recent, representative and periodic data for both adults and youth

SMOKE-FREE POLICIES: POLICIES ON SMOKE-FREE ENVIRONMENTS

	Data not reported
	Up to two public places completely smoke-free
	Three to five public places completely smoke-free
	Six to seven public places completely smoke-free
	All public places completely smoke-free (or at least 90% of the population covered by complete subnational smoke-free legislation)

CESSATION PROGRAMMES: TREATMENT OF TOBACCO DEPENDENCE

	Data not reported
	None
	NRT and/or some cessation services (neither cost-covered)
	NRT and/or some cessation services (at least one of which is cost-covered)
	National quit line, and both NRT and some cessation services cost-covered

WARNINGS: HEALTH WARNINGS ON CIGARETTE PACKAGES

	Data not reported
	No warnings or small warnings
	Medium size warnings missing some appropriate characteristics OR large warnings missing many appropriate characteristics
	Medium size warnings with all appropriate characteristics OR large warnings missing some appropriate characteristics
	Large warnings with all appropriate characteristics

WARNINGS: ANTI-TOBACCO MASS MEDIA CAMPAIGNS

	Data not reported
	No campaign conducted between January 2009 and August 2010 with duration of at least three weeks
	Campaign conducted with 1–4 appropriate characteristics
	Campaign conducted with 5–6 appropriate characteristics
	Campaign conducted with all appropriate characteristics

ADVERTISING BANS: BANS ON ADVERTISING, PROMOTION AND SPONSORSHIP

	Data not reported
	Complete absence of ban, or ban that does not cover national television, radio and print media
	Ban on national television, radio and print media only
	Ban on national television, radio and print media as well as on some but not all other forms of direct and/or indirect advertising
	Ban on all forms of direct and indirect advertising

TAXATION: SHARE OF TOTAL TAXES IN THE RETAIL PRICE OF THE MOST WIDELY SOLD BRAND OF CIGARETTES

	Data not reported
	≤ 25% of retail price is tax
	26–50% of retail price is tax
	51–75% of retail price is tax
	>75% of retail price is tax

COMPLIANCE: COMPLIANCE WITH BANS ON ADVERTISING, PROMOTION AND SPONSORSHIP, AND ADHERENCE TO SMOKE-FREE POLICY

									Complete compliance (8/10 to 10/10)
			Moderate compliance (3/10 to 7/10)
	Minimal compliance (0/10 to 2/10)

SYMBOLS LEGEND

»	Data not substantiated by a copy of the legislation
☉	Policy adopted but not implemented by 31 December 2010
▲ ▼	Change in POWER indicator group, up or down, between 2008 and 2010. Some 2008 data were revised in 2010. 2010 grouping rules were applied to both years

Refer to Technical Note I
for definitions of categories

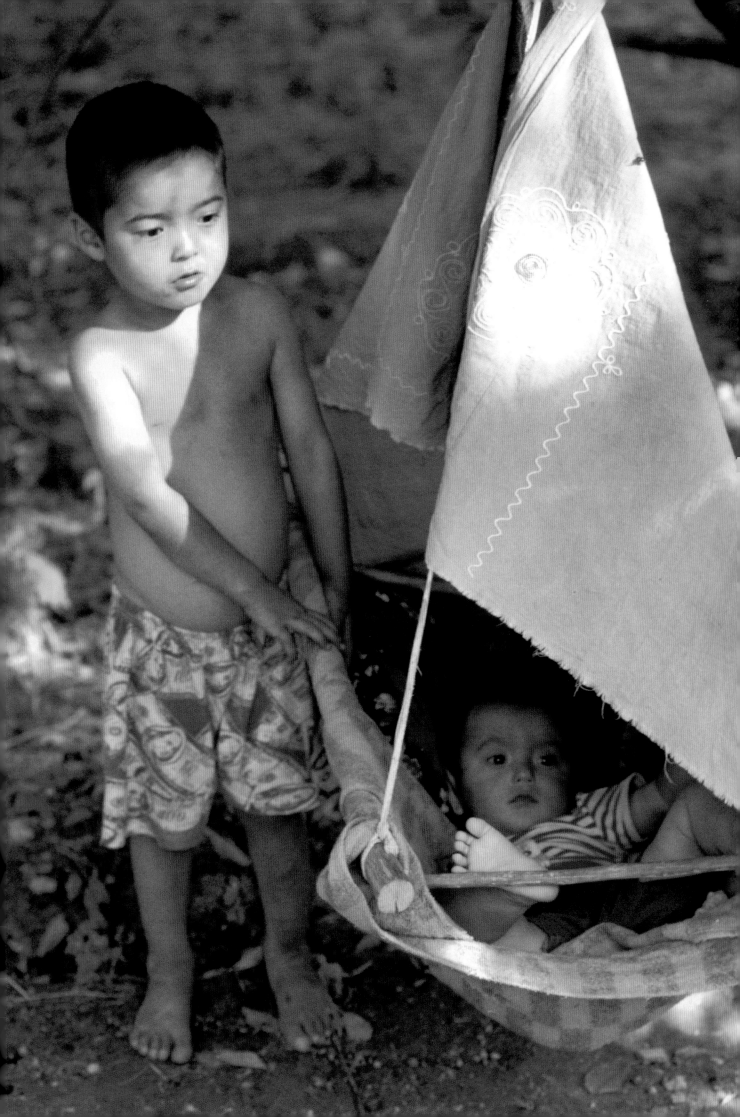

APPENDIX II: REGULATION OF WARNING LABELS ON CIGARETTE PACKAGES AND NATIONAL ANTI–TOBACCO MASS MEDIA CAMPAIGNS

Appendix II provides detailed information on legislation for warning labels on tobacco products and on anti-tobacco mass media campaigns in Member States. Data are provided for each WHO region.

Data on health warnings were primarily drawn from supporting legal documents such as adopted legislation and regulations. Available documents were reviewed by WHO and discussed with countries as necessary to ensure the correct interpretation. Data on anti-tobacco mass media campaigns were obtained from Member States directly.

Africa

Table 2.1.1
Characteristics* of health warning labels on cigarette packages in Africa

Please refer to page 118 for country-specific notes.

* Characteristics used to construct the categories for this report are described in Technical Note I.
» Data not substantiated by a copy of the legislation.
... Data not reported/not available.
— Data not required/not applicable.
^ Not mandated.

COUNTRY	HEALTH WARNING LABELS MANDATED	PERCENTAGE OF PRINCIPAL DISPLAY AREA MANDATED TO BE COVERED BY HEALTH WARNINGS		
		AVERAGE OF FRONT AND BACK %	FRONT %	BACK %
Algeria	Yes	15	15	15
Angola	No	—	—	—
Benin	Yes	30	30	30
Botswana	No	—	—	—
Burkina Faso[1]	Yes	—	—	—
Burundi	...	...	...	...
Cameroon	Yes	50	50	50
Cape Verde	Yes	^	^	^
Central African Republic	No	—	—	—
Chad	Yes	50	50	50
Comoros	No	—	—	—
Congo	No	—	—	—
Côte d'Ivoire	Yes	^	^	^
Democratic Republic of the Congo	Yes	30	30	30
Equatorial Guinea	No	—	—	—
Eritrea	Yes	50	50	50
Ethiopia	No	—	—	—
Gabon	No	—	—	—
Gambia	Yes	30	30	30
Ghana	Yes	5	—	—
Guinea	Yes	^	^	^
Guinea-Bissau*	Yes	—	45	—
Kenya	Yes	40	30	50
Lesotho	...	...	...	...
Liberia	No	—	—	—
Madagascar	Yes	50	50	50
Malawi	No	—	—	—
Mali	Yes	^	^	^
Mauritania	No	—	—	—
Mauritius	Yes	65	60	70
Mozambique	Yes	28	30	25
Namibia	Yes	^	^	^
Niger	Yes	30	30	30
Nigeria	Yes	^	^	^
Rwanda	No	—	—	—
Sao Tome and Principe	No	—	—	—
Senegal	Yes	^	^	^
Seychelles	Yes	50	—	—
Sierra Leone	No	—	—	—
South Africa	Yes	20	15	25
Swaziland	Yes	^	^	^
Togo	No	—	—	—
Uganda	No	—	—	—
United Republic of Tanzania	Yes	^	^	^
Zambia	Yes	^	^	^
Zimbabwe	Yes	20	15	25

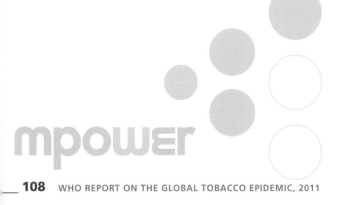

mpower

			SPECIFIC HEALTH WARNING LABELS ON PACKAGES				
DOES THE LAW MANDATE SPECIFIC HEALTH WARNINGS ON PACKAGES?	HOW MANY HEALTH WARNINGS ARE APPROVED BY THE LAW?	DO HEALTH WARNINGS APPEAR ON EACH PACKAGE AND ANY OUTSIDE PACKAGING AND LABELLING USED IN RETAIL SALE?	DO HEALTH WARNINGS DESCRIBE THE HARMFUL EFFECTS OF TOBACCO USE ON HEALTH?	DOES THE LAW MANDATE FONT STYLE, FONT SIZE AND COLOUR OF HEALTH WARNINGS?	ARE THE HEALTH WARNINGS ROTATING?	ARE THE HEALTH WARNINGS WRITTEN IN THE PRINCIPAL LANGUAGE(S) OF THE COUNTRY?	DO THE HEALTH WARNINGS INCLUDE A PHOTOGRAPH OR GRAPHIC?
Yes	6	No	Yes	No	Yes	Yes	No
—	—	—	—	—	—	—	—
Yes	1	Yes	No	No	No	No	No
—	—	—	—	—	—	—	—
Yes	1	No	No	No	No	No	No
…	…	…	…	…	…	…	…
Yes	1	Yes	Yes	Yes	No	Yes	No
No	—	No	No	No	No	No	No
—	—	—	—	—	—	—	—
No	—	Yes	No	No	No	No	No
—	—	—	—	—	—	—	—
—	—	—	—	—	—	—	—
Yes	1	Yes	No	No	No	Yes	No
Yes	4	Yes	Yes	Yes	No	No	No
—	—	—	—	—	—	—	—
Yes	5	Yes	Yes	No	Yes	Yes	No
—	—	—	—	—	—	—	—
—	—	—	—	—	—	—	—
Yes	2	Yes	Yes	No	No	No	No
Yes	1	No	No	No	No	No	No
Yes	1	No	Yes	No	No	No	No
No	—	No	No	No	No	No	No
Yes	14	No	Yes	Yes	Yes	Yes	No
…	…	…	…	…	…	…	…
—	—	—	—	—	—	—	—
Yes	1	Yes	Yes	No	No	Yes	No
—	—	—	—	—	—	—	—
Yes	1	Yes	Yes	No	No	Yes	No
—	—	—	—	—	—	—	—
Yes	8	Yes	Yes	Yes	Yes	Yes	Yes
No	—	Yes	Yes	No	No	Yes	No
No	—	No	Yes	No	No	No	No
Yes	1	Yes	No	No	No	No	No
Yes	2	Yes	Yes	No	Yes	Yes	No
—	—	—	—	—	—	—	—
—	—	—	—	—	—	—	—
Yes	1	Yes	No	No	No	Yes	No
No	—	Yes	No	No	No	Yes	No
—	—	—	—	—	—	—	—
Yes	8	Yes	Yes	Yes	Yes	Yes	No
—	—	Yes	Yes	—	—	—	—
—	—	—	—	—	—	—	—
No	—	No	No	No	No	No	No
Yes	10	No	Yes	No	No	Yes	No
Yes	1	Yes	No	No	No	No	No
Yes	1	Yes	Yes	Yes	No	No	No

The Americas

Table 2.1.2
Characteristics* of health warning labels on cigarette packages in the Americas

Please refer to page 118 for country-specific notes.

* Characteristics used to construct the categories for this report are described in Technical Note I.

⊙ Policy adopted but not implemented by 31 December 2010.

— Data not required/not applicable.

∧ Not mandated.

COUNTRY	HEALTH WARNING LABELS MANDATED	PERCENTAGE OF PRINCIPAL DISPLAY AREA MANDATED TO BE COVERED BY HEALTH WARNINGS		
		AVERAGE OF FRONT AND BACK %	FRONT %	BACK %
Antigua and Barbuda	No	—	—	—
Argentina	Yes	∧	∧	∧
Bahamas	Yes	∧	∧	∧
Barbados	No	—	—	—
Belize	No	—	—	—
Bolivia (Plurinational State of)	Yes	50	50	50
Brazil	Yes	50	0	100
Canada	Yes	50	50	50
Chile	Yes	50	50	50
Colombia	Yes	30	30	30
Costa Rica	Yes	∧	∧	∧
Cuba	Yes	30	30	30
Dominica	No	—	—	—
Dominican Republic	Yes	∧	∧	∧
Ecuador	Yes	40	40	40
El Salvador	Yes	∧	∧	∧
Grenada	No	—	—	—
Guatemala	Yes	13	25	0
Guyana	Yes	∧	∧	∧
Haiti	No	—	—	—
Honduras	Yes ⊙	80²	80²	80²
Jamaica	Yes	30	30	30
Mexico	Yes	65	30	100
Nicaragua	Yes ⊙	50 ⊙	50 ⊙	50 ⊙
Panama	Yes	50	50	50
Paraguay	Yes	∧	∧	∧
Peru	Yes	50 ⊙	50 ⊙	50 ⊙
Saint Kitts and Nevis	No	—	—	—
Saint Lucia	No	—	—	—
Saint Vincent and the Grenadines	No	—	—	—
Suriname	No	—	—	—
Trinidad and Tobago	Yes ⊙	∧³	∧³	∧³
United States of America	Yes ⊙	50 ⊙	50 ⊙	50 ⊙
Uruguay	Yes	80	80	80
Venezuela (Bolivarian Republic of)	Yes	50	0	100

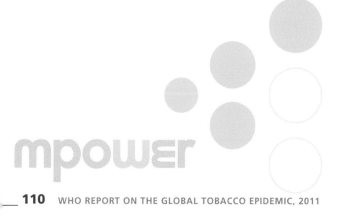

mpower

SPECIFIC HEALTH WARNING LABELS ON PACKAGES

DOES THE LAW MANDATE SPECIFIC HEALTH WARNINGS ON PACKAGES?	HOW MANY HEALTH WARNINGS ARE APPROVED BY THE LAW?	DO HEALTH WARNINGS APPEAR ON EACH PACKAGE AND ANY OUTSIDE PACKAGING AND LABELLING USED IN RETAIL SALE?	DO HEALTH WARNINGS DESCRIBE THE HARMFUL EFFECTS OF TOBACCO USE ON HEALTH?	DOES THE LAW MANDATE FONT STYLE, FONT SIZE AND COLOUR OF HEALTH WARNINGS?	ARE THE HEALTH WARNINGS ROTATING?	ARE THE HEALTH WARNINGS WRITTEN IN THE PRINCIPAL LANGUAGE(S) OF THE COUNTRY?	DO THE HEALTH WARNINGS INCLUDE A PHOTOGRAPH OR GRAPHIC?
—	—	—	—	—	—	—	—
Yes	1	Yes	No	No	No	Yes	No
Yes	1	Yes	Yes	No	No	Yes	No
—	—	—	—	—	—	—	—
—	—	—	—	—	—	—	—
Yes	6	Yes	Yes	Yes	Yes	Yes	Yes
Yes	10	Yes	Yes	Yes	Yes	Yes	Yes
Yes	16	Yes	Yes	Yes	No	Yes	Yes
Yes	1	Yes	Yes	Yes	Yes	Yes	Yes
Yes	6	Yes	Yes	Yes	Yes	Yes	Yes
Yes	2	Yes	Yes	No	Yes	Yes	No
Yes	5	Yes	Yes	Yes	Yes	Yes	No
—	—	—	—	—	—	—	—
Yes	1	Yes	No	Yes	No	Yes	No
Yes	3	Yes	Yes	Yes	No	Yes	No
Yes	1	Yes	No	No	No	Yes	No
—	—	—	—	—	—	—	—
Yes	6	Yes	Yes	Yes	Yes	Yes	No
Yes	1	Yes	No	Yes	No	Yes	No
—	—	—	—	—	—	—	—
No[3]	—	Yes $\circ$	No[3]	No[3]	Yes $\circ$	Yes $\circ$	Yes $\circ$
Yes	12	Yes	Yes	Yes	Yes	Yes	No
Yes	8	Yes	Yes	Yes	Yes	Yes	Yes
Yes $\circ$	6 $\circ$	Yes $\circ$	No[3]	Yes $\circ$	Yes $\circ$	Yes $\circ$	Yes $\circ$
Yes	5	Yes	Yes	Yes	Yes	Yes	Yes
Yes	1	Yes	No	No	No	Yes	No
Yes	11	Yes	Yes	Yes	Yes	Yes	Yes
—	—	—	—	—	—	—	—
—	—	—	—	—	—	—	—
—	—	—	—	—	—	—	—
—	—	—	—	—	—	—	—
Yes $\circ$	$\wedge$[3]	Yes $\circ$	No	Yes $\circ$	No	Yes $\circ$	No
Yes $\circ$	9 $\circ$	Yes $\circ$	Yes $\circ$	Yes $\circ$	Yes $\circ$	Yes $\circ$	Yes $\circ$
Yes	6	Yes	Yes	Yes	Yes	Yes	Yes
Yes	10	Yes	Yes	Yes	Yes	Yes	Yes

South-East Asia

Table 2.1.3
Characteristics* of health warning labels on cigarette packages in South-East Asia

Please refer to page 118 for country-specific notes.

* Characteristics used to construct the categories for this report are described in Technical Note I.
... Data not reported/not available.
— Data not required/not applicable.
^ Not mandated.
⊙ Policy adopted but not implemented by 31 December 2010.

COUNTRY	HEALTH WARNING LABELS MANDATED	PERCENTAGE OF PRINCIPAL DISPLAY AREA MANDATED TO BE COVERED BY HEALTH WARNINGS		
		AVERAGE OF FRONT AND BACK %	FRONT %	BACK %
Bangladesh	Yes	30	30	30
Bhutan [4]	Yes	^	^	^
Democratic People's Republic of Korea	Yes	^	^	^
India	Yes	20	40	0
Indonesia	Yes	^	^	^
Maldives	Yes	30	30	30
Myanmar	Yes	^	^	^
Nepal	Yes	15	30	0
Sri Lanka	Yes	^	^	^
Thailand	Yes	55	55	55
Timor-Leste	Yes	^	^	^

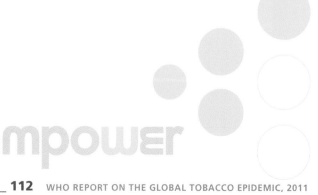

mpower

			SPECIFIC HEALTH WARNING LABELS ON PACKAGES				
DOES THE LAW MANDATE SPECIFIC HEALTH WARNINGS ON PACKAGES?	HOW MANY HEALTH WARNINGS ARE APPROVED BY THE LAW?	DO HEALTH WARNINGS APPEAR ON EACH PACKAGE AND ANY OUTSIDE PACKAGING AND LABELLING USED IN RETAIL SALE?	DO HEALTH WARNINGS DESCRIBE THE HARMFUL EFFECTS OF TOBACCO USE ON HEALTH?	DOES THE LAW MANDATE FONT STYLE, FONT SIZE AND COLOUR OF HEALTH WARNINGS?	ARE THE HEALTH WARNINGS ROTATING?	ARE THE HEALTH WARNINGS WRITTEN IN THE PRINCIPAL LANGUAGE(S) OF THE COUNTRY?	DO THE HEALTH WARNINGS INCLUDE A PHOTOGRAPH OR GRAPHIC?
Yes	6	Yes	Yes	Yes	Yes	Yes	No
No	—	No	No	No	No	No	No
Yes	1	No	Yes	No	No	No	No
Yes	2	Yes	Yes	Yes	Yes	Yes	Yes
Yes	1	Yes	Yes	No	No	Yes	No
Yes	5	Yes ⁰	Yes	No	Yes	Yes ⁰	No
Yes	. . .	No	No	No	No	Yes	No
No	—	Yes	No	No	Yes	Yes	Yes
Yes	2	No	Yes	No	No	No	No
Yes	10	Yes	Yes	Yes	Yes	Yes	Yes
Yes	5	No	Yes	No	No	Yes	No

Europe

Table 2.1.4
Characteristics* of health warning labels on cigarette packages in Europe

Please refer to page 118 for country-specific notes.

* Characteristics used to construct the categories for this report are described in Technical Note I.

⊙ Policy adopted but not implemented by 31 December 2010.

... Data not reported/not available.

— Data not required/not applicable.

^ Not mandated.

COUNTRY	HEALTH WARNING LABELS MANDATED	PERCENTAGE OF PRINCIPAL DISPLAY AREA MANDATED TO BE COVERED BY HEALTH WARNINGS		
		AVERAGE OF FRONT AND BACK %	FRONT %	BACK %
Albania	Yes	50	50	50
Andorra[5]	...	...	...	...
Armenia	Yes	30	30	30
Austria	Yes	35	30	40
Azerbaijan	Yes	^	^	^
Belarus	Yes	30	30	30
Belgium	Yes	43	35	50
Bosnia and Herzegovina[6]	...	...	...	...
Bulgaria	Yes	35	30	40
Croatia	Yes	35	30	40
Cyprus	Yes	39	32	45
Czech Republic	Yes	35	30	40
Denmark	Yes	35	30	40
Estonia	Yes	35	30	40
Finland	Yes	39	32	45
France	Yes	35	30	40
Georgia	Yes	30	30	30
Germany	Yes	35	30	40
Greece	Yes	35	30	40
Hungary	Yes	35	30	40
Iceland	Yes	35	30	40
Ireland	Yes	39	32	45
Israel	Yes	30	30	30
Italy	Yes	35	30	40
Kazakhstan	Yes	40	0	40
Kyrgyzstan	Yes	40	40	40
Latvia	Yes	35	30	40
Lithuania	Yes	35	30	40
Luxembourg	Yes	39	32	45
Malta	Yes	39	32	45
Monaco[7]	...	...	...	...
Montenegro	Yes	35	30	40
Netherlands	Yes	35	30	40
Norway	Yes	35	30	40
Poland	Yes	35	30	40
Portugal	Yes	35	30	40
Republic of Moldova	Yes	35	30	40
Romania	Yes	35	30	40
Russian Federation	Yes	40	30	50
San Marino	No	—	—	—
Serbia	Yes	35	30	40
Slovakia	Yes	35	30	40
Slovenia	Yes	35	30	40
Spain	Yes	35	30	40
Sweden	Yes	35	30	40
Switzerland	Yes	43	35	50
Tajikistan	No	—	—	—
The former Yugoslav Republic of Macedonia	Yes	35	30	40
Turkey	Yes	48	30	65
Turkmenistan	No	—	—	—
Ukraine	Yes ⊙	50 ⊙	50 ⊙	50 ⊙
United Kingdom of Great Britain and Northern Ireland	Yes	35	30	40
Uzbekistan	Yes	30	30	30

mpower

SPECIFIC HEALTH WARNING LABELS ON PACKAGES							
DOES THE LAW MANDATE SPECIFIC HEALTH WARNINGS ON PACKAGES?	HOW MANY HEALTH WARNINGS ARE APPROVED BY THE LAW?	DO HEALTH WARNINGS APPEAR ON EACH PACKAGE AND ANY OUTSIDE PACKAGING AND LABELLING USED IN RETAIL SALE?	DO HEALTH WARNINGS DESCRIBE THE HARMFUL EFFECTS OF TOBACCO USE ON HEALTH?	DOES THE LAW MANDATE FONT STYLE, FONT SIZE AND COLOUR OF HEALTH WARNINGS?	ARE THE HEALTH WARNINGS ROTATING?	ARE THE HEALTH WARNINGS WRITTEN IN THE PRINCIPAL LANGUAGE(S) OF THE COUNTRY?	DO THE HEALTH WARNINGS INCLUDE A PHOTOGRAPH OR GRAPHIC?
Yes	16	Yes	Yes	Yes	Yes	Yes	No
...	...	...	...	...	...	...	...
Yes	5	Yes	Yes	Yes	Yes	Yes	No
Yes	16	Yes	Yes	Yes	Yes	Yes	No
No	—	No	No	No	No	Yes	No
Yes	6	Yes	Yes	No	Yes	Yes	No
Yes	16	Yes	Yes	Yes	Yes	Yes	Yes
...	...	...	...	...	...	...	...
Yes	16	Yes	Yes	Yes	Yes	Yes	No
Yes	16	No	Yes	Yes	Yes	Yes	No
Yes	13	Yes	Yes	Yes	Yes	Yes	No
Yes	16	Yes	Yes	Yes	Yes	Yes	No
Yes	16	Yes	Yes	Yes	Yes	Yes	No
Yes	16	Yes	Yes	Yes	Yes	Yes	No
Yes	16	Yes	Yes	Yes	Yes	Yes	No
Yes	16	Yes	Yes	Yes	Yes	Yes	Yes
Yes	12	Yes	Yes	Yes	Yes	Yes	Yes
Yes	16	Yes	Yes	Yes	Yes	Yes	No
Yes	16	Yes	Yes	Yes	Yes	Yes	No
Yes	16	Yes	Yes	Yes	Yes	Yes	No
Yes	16	Yes	Yes	Yes	Yes	Yes	No
Yes	16	Yes	Yes	Yes	Yes	Yes	No
Yes	13	Yes	Yes	Yes	Yes	Yes	No
Yes	10	Yes	Yes	Yes	Yes	Yes	No
No	—	No	No	No	No	No	No
Yes	9	Yes	Yes	Yes	Yes	Yes	No
Yes	16	Yes	Yes	Yes	Yes	Yes	Yes
Yes	16	Yes	Yes	Yes	Yes	Yes	No
Yes	17	Yes	Yes	No	Yes	Yes	No
Yes	16	Yes	Yes	Yes	Yes	Yes	Yes °
...	...	...	...	...	...	...	...
Yes	16	Yes	Yes	Yes	Yes	Yes	No
Yes	16	Yes	Yes	Yes	Yes	Yes	No
Yes	16	Yes	Yes	Yes	Yes	Yes	Yes °
Yes	16	Yes	Yes	Yes	Yes	Yes	No
Yes	16	Yes	Yes	Yes	Yes	Yes	No
Yes	14	Yes	Yes	Yes	Yes	Yes	No
Yes	16	Yes	Yes	Yes	Yes	Yes	Yes
Yes	13	No	Yes	No	Yes	Yes	No
—	—	—	—	—	—	—	—
Yes	12	Yes	Yes	Yes	Yes	Yes	No
Yes	16	Yes	Yes	Yes	Yes	Yes	No
Yes	16	Yes	Yes	Yes	Yes	Yes	No
Yes	16	Yes	Yes	Yes	Yes	Yes	Yes
Yes	14	Yes	Yes	Yes	Yes	Yes	No
Yes	16	Yes	Yes	No	Yes	Yes	Yes
—	—	—	—	—	—	—	—
Yes	16	Yes	Yes	Yes	Yes	Yes	Yes
Yes	16	Yes	Yes	Yes	Yes	Yes	Yes
—	—	—	—	—	—	—	—
Yes °	10 °	Yes °	Yes °	No	Yes °	Yes °	Yes °
Yes	16	Yes	Yes	Yes	Yes	Yes	Yes
Yes	3	No	Yes	No	Yes	Yes	No

Eastern Mediterranean

Table 2.1.5
Characteristics* of health warning labels on cigarette packages in the Eastern Mediterranean

Please refer to page 118 for country-specific notes.

* Characteristics used to construct the categories for this report are described in Technical Note I.
... Data not reported/not available.
— Data not required/not applicable.
^ Not mandated.
< Refers to a territory.

COUNTRY	HEALTH WARNING LABELS MANDATED	PERCENTAGE OF PRINCIPAL DISPLAY AREA MANDATED TO BE COVERED BY HEALTH WARNINGS		
		AVERAGE OF FRONT AND BACK %	FRONT %	BACK %
Afghanistan	No	—	—	—
Bahrain	Yes	^	^	^
Djibouti	Yes	50	50	50
Egypt	Yes	50	50	50
Iran (Islamic Republic of)	Yes	50	50	50
Iraq	Yes	...	...	...
Jordan	Yes	30	30	30
Kuwait	Yes	^	^	^
Lebanon	Yes	15	15	15
Libyan Arab Jamahiriya	Yes	25	50	0
Morocco	Yes	^	^	^
Oman	Yes	^	^	^
Pakistan	Yes	40	40	40
Qatar	Yes	^8	^8	^8
Saudi Arabia	Yes	^	^	^
Somalia	No	—	—	—
Sudan	Yes	15	30	0
Syrian Arab Republic	Yes	15	30	0
Tunisia	Yes	^	^	^
United Arab Emirates	Yes	^	^	^
West Bank and Gaza Strip<	Yes	10	20	0
Yemen	Yes	33	—	—

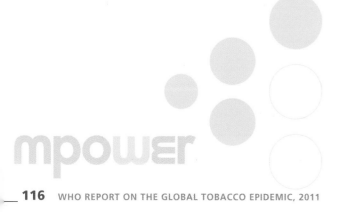

			SPECIFIC HEALTH WARNING LABELS ON PACKAGES				
DOES THE LAW MANDATE SPECIFIC HEALTH WARNINGS ON PACKAGES?	HOW MANY HEALTH WARNINGS ARE APPROVED BY THE LAW?	DO HEALTH WARNINGS APPEAR ON EACH PACKAGE AND ANY OUTSIDE PACKAGING AND LABELLING USED IN RETAIL SALE?	DO HEALTH WARNINGS DESCRIBE THE HARMFUL EFFECTS OF TOBACCO USE ON HEALTH?	DOES THE LAW MANDATE FONT STYLE, FONT SIZE AND COLOUR OF HEALTH WARNINGS?	ARE THE HEALTH WARNINGS ROTATING?	ARE THE HEALTH WARNINGS WRITTEN IN THE PRINCIPAL LANGUAGE(S) OF THE COUNTRY?	DO THE HEALTH WARNINGS INCLUDE A PHOTOGRAPH OR GRAPHIC?
—	—	—	—	—	—	—	—
No	—	Yes	No	No	No	Yes	No
Yes	16	Yes	Yes	Yes	Yes	Yes	Yes
Yes	8	Yes	Yes	Yes	Yes	Yes	Yes
Yes	8	Yes	Yes	Yes	Yes	Yes	Yes
No	—	No	Yes	No	No	Yes	No
Yes	1	Yes	Yes	Yes	No	Yes	Yes
Yes	1	Yes	Yes	Yes	No	Yes	No
Yes	1	Yes	Yes	No	No	Yes	No
Yes	1	Yes	Yes	No	Yes	Yes	No
Yes	1	No	No	No	No	No	No
No	—	Yes	No	No	No	Yes	No
Yes	1	Yes	Yes	Yes	Yes	Yes	Yes
Yes	1	Yes	Yes	Yes	No	Yes	No
Yes	1	No	Yes	No	No	Yes	No
—	—	—	—	—	—	—	—
Yes	1	No	Yes	No	Yes	Yes	No
Yes	1	Yes	Yes	No	No	Yes	No
Yes	1	Yes	Yes	No	No	Yes	No
No	—	Yes	Yes	No	Yes	No	Yes
No	—	Yes	Yes	No	No	No	No
No	—	Yes	Yes	No	No	Yes	No

Western Pacific

Table 2.1.6
Characteristics* of health warning labels on cigarette packages in the Western Pacific

* Characteristics used to construct the categories for this report are described in Technical Note I.

⊙ Policy adopted but not implemented by 31 December 2010.

... Data not reported/not available.

— Data not required/not applicable.

∧ Not mandated.

NOTES TO APPENDIX II TABLE 2.1

1. Regulations will be issued shortly.
2. The law was adopted in August 2010 and was scheduled to enter into force in February 2011. However, the law was amended in April 2011, mandating a size of 50% on the front and back of the package.
3. Regulations pending.
4. Bhutan prohibits the sale of all tobacco products; tobacco products imported for personal consumption shall show the country of origin and appropriate health warnings as required by the Ministry of Health.
5. All tobacco products sold in Andorra are imported from France or Spain and therefore follow the French or Spanish laws on health warnings.
6. The two subnational jurisdictions of the country, Federation of Bosnia and Herzegovina and Republika Srpska, adopted separate tobacco control legislation with several differences, so no national legislation is reported.
7. All tobacco products sold in Monaco are imported from France and therefore follow the French law on health warnings.
8. At least 25% of the surface occupied by the trademark is mandated for the health warning; in practice the size of the warning is less than 30% of the package.

COUNTRY	HEALTH WARNING LABELS MANDATED	PERCENTAGE OF PRINCIPAL DISPLAY AREA MANDATED TO BE COVERED BY HEALTH WARNINGS		
		AVERAGE OF FRONT AND BACK %	FRONT %	BACK %
Australia	Yes	60	30	90
Brunei Darussalam	Yes	50	50	50
Cambodia	Yes	30	30	30
China	Yes	30	30	30
Cook Islands	Yes	50	50	50
Fiji	Yes	20	—	—
Japan	Yes	30	30	30
Kiribati	...	...	...	...
Lao People's Democratic Republic	Yes	30	30	30
Malaysia	Yes	50	40	60
Marshall Islands	Yes	∧	∧	∧
Micronesia (Federated States of)	No	—	—	—
Mongolia	Yes	33	33	33
Nauru	Yes	13	0	25
New Zealand	Yes	60	30	90
Niue	No	—	—	—
Palau	No	—	—	—
Papua New Guinea	Yes	∧	∧	∧
Philippines	Yes	45	30	60
Republic of Korea	Yes	30	30	30
Samoa	Yes	30	30	30
Singapore	Yes	50	50	50
Solomon Islands	Yes ⊙	30 ⊙	—	—
Tonga	Yes	30	30	30
Tuvalu	Yes	30	30	30
Vanuatu	Yes	30	—	—
Viet Nam	Yes	30	30	30

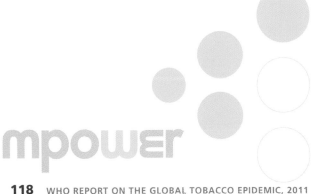

			SPECIFIC HEALTH WARNING LABELS ON PACKAGES				
DOES THE LAW MANDATE SPECIFIC HEALTH WARNINGS ON PACKAGES?	HOW MANY HEALTH WARNINGS ARE APPROVED BY THE LAW?	DO HEALTH WARNINGS APPEAR ON EACH PACKAGE AND ANY OUTSIDE PACKAGING AND LABELLING USED IN RETAIL SALE?	DO HEALTH WARNINGS DESCRIBE THE HARMFUL EFFECTS OF TOBACCO USE ON HEALTH?	DOES THE LAW MANDATE FONT STYLE, FONT SIZE AND COLOUR OF HEALTH WARNINGS?	ARE THE HEALTH WARNINGS ROTATING?	ARE THE HEALTH WARNINGS WRITTEN IN THE PRINCIPAL LANGUAGE(S) OF THE COUNTRY?	DO THE HEALTH WARNINGS INCLUDE A PHOTOGRAPH OR GRAPHIC?
Yes	14	Yes	Yes	Yes	Yes	Yes	Yes
Yes	6	Yes	Yes	Yes	Yes	Yes	Yes
Yes	5	No	Yes	Yes	No	Yes	No
Yes	3	Yes	Yes	Yes	Yes	Yes	No
Yes	14	Yes	Yes	Yes	Yes	Yes	No
No	—	Yes	No	No	No	No	No
Yes	8	Yes	Yes	Yes	Yes	Yes	No
...	...	...	...	...	...	...	...
Yes	6	Yes	Yes	Yes	Yes	Yes	No
Yes	6	Yes	Yes	Yes	Yes	Yes	Yes
No	—	Yes	Yes	No	No	No	No
—	—	—	—	—	—	—	—
Yes	6	Yes	Yes	Yes	Yes	Yes	Yes
Yes	6	Yes	Yes	Yes	Yes	Yes	No
Yes	14	Yes	Yes	Yes	Yes	Yes	Yes
—	—	—	—	—	—	—	—
—	—	—	—	—	—	—	—
...	3	Yes	...	...	...	...	...
Yes	4	Yes	Yes	Yes	Yes	Yes	No
Yes	3	Yes	Yes	No	Yes	Yes	No
No	—	Yes	No	No	Yes	No	No
Yes	6	Yes	Yes	Yes	Yes	Yes	Yes
No	—	Yes ⊗	Yes ⊗	No	Yes ⊗	Yes ⊗	No
No	—	Yes	No	No	Yes	Yes	No
Yes	6	Yes	Yes	Yes	Yes	No	No
Yes	4	Yes	Yes	No	Yes	Yes	No
Yes	2	Yes	Yes	No	Yes	Yes	No

Africa

Table 2.2.1
Additional characteristics of health warning labels on cigarette packages in Africa

Please refer to page 130 for country-specific notes.

* Terms including, but not limited to, "low tar", "light", "ultra light" or "mild", in any language.

. . . Data not reported/not available.

COUNTRY	OTHER REQUIREMENTS FOR HEALTH WARNING LABELS ON PACKAGES		
	WARNING MUST BE PLACED AT THE TOP OF THE PRINCIPAL DISPLAY AREA	WARNINGS MUST NOT REMOVE OR DIMINISH THE LIABILITY OF THE TOBACCO INDUSTRY	LAW APPLIES TO PRODUCTS WHETHER MANUFACTURED DOMESTICALLY, IMPORTED, OR FOR DUTY-FREE SALE
Algeria	No	No	Yes
Angola	No	No	No
Benin	No	No	Yes
Botswana	No	No	No
Burkina Faso[1]	No	No	Yes
Burundi	. . .	. . .	. . .
Cameroon	No	No	Yes
Cape Verde	No	No	Yes
Central African Republic	No	No	No
Chad	No	No	Yes
Comoros	No	No	No
Congo	No	No	No
Côte d'Ivoire	No	No	Yes
Democratic Republic of the Congo	No	No	Yes
Equatorial Guinea	No	No	No
Eritrea	No	Yes	Yes
Ethiopia	No	No	No
Gabon	No	No	No
Gambia	No	No	No
Ghana	No	No	Yes
Guinea	No	No	Yes
Guinea-Bissau	. . .	. . .	. . .
Kenya	No	No	Yes
Lesotho	. . .	. . .	. . .
Liberia	No	No	No
Madagascar	No	No	Yes
Malawi	No	No	No
Mali	No	No	No
Mauritania	No	No	No
Mauritius	No	No	Yes
Mozambique	No	No	Yes
Namibia	No	No	Yes
Niger	No	No	Yes
Nigeria	No	No	Yes
Rwanda	No	No	No
Sao Tome and Principe	No	No	No
Senegal	No	No	No
Seychelles	No	No	Yes
Sierra Leone	No	No	No
South Africa	Yes	Yes	Yes
Swaziland	No	No	Yes
Togo	No	No	No
Uganda	No	No	No
United Republic of Tanzania	No	No	Yes
Zambia	No	No	Yes
Zimbabwe	Yes	No	Yes

mpower

OTHER REQUIREMENTS FOR HEALTH WARNING LABELS ON PACKAGES		OTHER RESTRICTIONS REGARDING PACKAGING					
WARNINGS MUST NOT BE OBSCURED IN ANY WAY, INCLUDING BY REQUIRED MARKINGS SUCH AS TAX STAMPS	LAW REQUIRES OR ESTABLISHES FINES FOR VIOLATIONS OF THE HEALTH WARNINGS LAW	BAN ON DECEITFUL TERMS*	BAN ON USE OF FIGURATIVE OR OTHER SIGNS, INCLUDING COLOURS OR NUMBERS	BAN ON PACKAGING AND LABELLING USING DESCRIPTORS DEPICTING FLAVOURS	BAN ON DISPLAY OF QUANTITATIVE INFORMATION ON EMISSION YIELDS (SUCH AS TAR, NICOTINE AND CARBON MONOXIDE)	QUIT LINE NUMBER REQUIRED TO APPEAR ON ALL PACKAGING OR LABELLING	DOES THE LAW MANDATE PLAIN PACKAGING?
No	No	No	No	No	No	No	No
No	No	...	...	...	...	...	...
No	Yes	No	No	No	No	No	No
No	No	No	No	No	No	No	No
No	Yes	No	No	No	No	No	No
...	...	...	...	...	...	...	...
No	Yes	No	No	No	No	No	No
No	Yes	No	No	No	No	No	No
No	No	No	No	No	No	No	No
No	Yes	No	No	No	No	No	No
No	No	...	...	...	...	...	...
No	No	...	...	...	...	...	...
Yes	Yes	No	No	No	No	No	No
No	Yes	No	No	No	No	No	No
No	No	...	...	...	...	...	...
No	Yes	Yes	Yes	No	No	No	No
No	No	No	No	No	No	No	No
No	No	No	No	No	Yes	No	No
No	No	No	No	No	No	No	No
No	No	No	No	No	No	No	No
No	Yes	No	No	No	No	No	No
...	...	...	...	...	...	...	...
No	Yes	Yes	Yes	No	No	No	No
...	...	...	...	...	...	...	...
No	No	No	No	No	No	No	No
No	No	No	No	No	No	No	No
No	No	No	No	No	No	No	No
No	Yes	Yes	Yes	No	Yes	No	No
No	No	No	No	No	No	No	No
Yes	Yes	Yes	No	No	Yes	No	No
No	No	Yes	Yes	No	No	No	No
No	Yes	No	No	No	No	No	No
No	Yes	Yes	Yes	No	No	No	No
No	Yes	No	No	No	No	No	No
No	No	No	No	No	No	No	No
No	No	No	No	No	No	No	No
No	Yes	No	No	No	No	No	No
No	Yes	Yes	Yes	No	No	No	No
No	No	...	...	...	...	...	...
Yes	Yes	Yes	Yes	No	No	Yes	No
No	Yes	Yes	No	No	No	No	No
No	No	...	...	...	...	...	...
No	No	No	No	No	No	No	No
No	Yes	Yes	No	No	No	No	No
No	No	No	No	No	No	No	No
No	Yes	No	No	No	No	No	No

The Americas

Table 2.2.2
Additional characteristics of health warning labels on cigarette packages in the Americas

* Terms including, but not limited to, "low tar", "light", "ultra light" or "mild", in any language.

⊙ Policy adopted but not implemented by 31 December 2010.

COUNTRY	OTHER REQUIREMENTS FOR HEALTH WARNING LABELS ON PACKAGES		
	WARNING MUST BE PLACED AT THE TOP OF THE PRINCIPAL DISPLAY AREA	WARNINGS MUST NOT REMOVE OR DIMINISH THE LIABILITY OF THE TOBACCO INDUSTRY	LAW APPLIES TO PRODUCTS WHETHER MANUFACTURED DOMESTICALLY, IMPORTED, OR FOR DUTY-FREE SALE
Antigua and Barbuda	No	No	No
Argentina	No	No	No
Bahamas	No	No	Yes
Barbados	No	No	No
Belize	No	No	No
Bolivia (Plurinational State of)	No	No	Yes
Brazil	Yes	No	Yes
Canada	Yes	Yes	Yes
Chile	No	No	Yes
Colombia	No	No	Yes
Costa Rica	No	No	No
Cuba	No	No	No
Dominica	No	No	No
Dominican Republic	No	No	No
Ecuador	No	No	No
El Salvador	No	No	No
Grenada	No	No	No
Guatemala	No	No	Yes
Guyana	No	No	No
Haiti	No	No	No
Honduras	No	Yes ⊙	Yes ⊙
Jamaica	No	No	No
Mexico	Yes	No	Yes
Nicaragua	No	No	No
Panama	No	Yes	Yes
Paraguay	No	No	No
Peru	No	No	No
Saint Kitts and Nevis	No	No	No
Saint Lucia	No	No	No
Saint Vincent and the Grenadines	No	No	No
Suriname	No	No	No
Trinidad and Tobago	No	No	Yes ⊙
United States of America	Yes ⊙	No	Yes
Uruguay	No	No	Yes
Venezuela (Bolivarian Republic of)	Yes	No	Yes

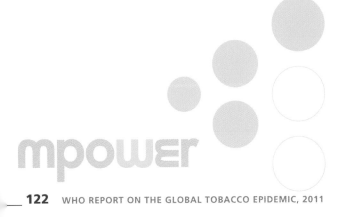

OTHER REQUIREMENTS FOR HEALTH WARNING LABELS ON PACKAGES		OTHER RESTRICTIONS REGARDING PACKAGING					
WARNINGS MUST NOT BE OBSCURED IN ANY WAY, INCLUDING BY REQUIRED MARKINGS SUCH AS TAX STAMPS	LAW REQUIRES OR ESTABLISHES FINES FOR VIOLATIONS OF THE HEALTH WARNINGS LAW	BAN ON DECEITFUL TERMS*	BAN ON USE OF FIGURATIVE OR OTHER SIGNS, INCLUDING COLOURS OR NUMBERS	BAN ON PACKAGING AND LABELLING USING DESCRIPTORS DEPICTING FLAVOURS	BAN ON DISPLAY OF QUANTITATIVE INFORMATION ON EMISSION YIELDS (SUCH AS TAR, NICOTINE AND CARBON MONOXIDE)	QUIT LINE NUMBER REQUIRED TO APPEAR ON ALL PACKAGING OR LABELLING	DOES THE LAW MANDATE PLAIN PACKAGING?
No	No	No	No	No	No	No	No
No	Yes	No	No	No	No	No	No
No	Yes	No	No	No	No	No	No
No	No	No	No	No	No	No	No
No	No	No	No	No	No	No	No
No	Yes	Yes	No	No	Yes	No	No
Yes	Yes	Yes	No	No	No	Yes	No
Yes	Yes	Yes	No	Yes	No	No	No
No	Yes	Yes	No	No	Yes	No	No
Yes	Yes	Yes	Yes	No	Yes	No	No
No	Yes	No	No	No	No	No	No
Yes	Yes	Yes	Yes	No	No	No	No
No	No	No	No	No	No	No	No
Yes	No	No	No	No	No	No	No
No	Yes	No	No	No	No	No	No
No	No	No	No	No	No	No	No
No	No	No	No	No	No	No	No
No	Yes	No	No	No	No	No	No
No	No	No	No	No	No	No	No
No	No	No	No	No	No	No	No
No	Yes °	Yes °	No	No	No	No	No
No	No	Yes	No	No	No	No	No
Yes	Yes	Yes	Yes	No	No	Yes	No
Yes °	Yes °	Yes °	No	No	No	No	No
Yes	Yes	Yes	Yes	Yes	Yes	No	No
No	Yes	No	No	No	No	No	No
No	Yes	Yes	No	No	No	No	No
No	No	No	No	No	No	No	No
No	No	No	No	No	No	No	No
No	No	No	No	No	No	No	No
No	No	No	No	No	No	No	No
Yes °	Yes °	Yes °	Yes °	No	No	No	No
No	Yes	Yes °	No	No	No	No	No
Yes	Yes	Yes	Yes	No	Yes	No	No
No	Yes	Yes	No	No	Yes	No	No

South-East Asia

Table 2.2.3
Additional characteristics of health warning labels on cigarette packages in South-East Asia

Please refer to page 130 for country-specific notes.

*   Terms including, but not limited to, "low tar", "light", "ultra light" or "mild", in any language.

⊙   Policy adopted but not implemented by 31 December 2010.

COUNTRY	OTHER REQUIREMENTS FOR HEALTH WARNING LABELS ON PACKAGES		
	WARNING MUST BE PLACED AT THE TOP OF THE PRINCIPAL DISPLAY AREA	WARNINGS MUST NOT REMOVE OR DIMINISH THE LIABILITY OF THE TOBACCO INDUSTRY	LAW APPLIES TO PRODUCTS WHETHER MANUFACTURED DOMESTICALLY, IMPORTED, OR FOR DUTY-FREE SALE
Bangladesh	Yes	No	Yes
Bhutan [2]	No	No	No
Democratic People's Republic of Korea	No	No	Yes
India	Yes	No	Yes
Indonesia	No	No	No
Maldives	No	Yes ⊙	Yes ⊙
Myanmar	No	No	No
Nepal	No	No	No
Sri Lanka	No	No	Yes
Thailand	Yes	No	No
Timor-Leste	No	No	Yes

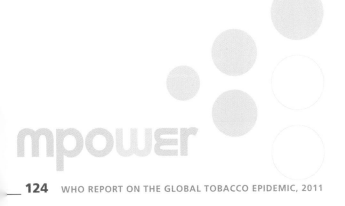

OTHER REQUIREMENTS FOR HEALTH WARNING LABELS ON PACKAGES		OTHER RESTRICTIONS REGARDING PACKAGING					
WARNINGS MUST NOT BE OBSCURED IN ANY WAY, INCLUDING BY REQUIRED MARKINGS SUCH AS TAX STAMPS	LAW REQUIRES OR ESTABLISHES FINES FOR VIOLATIONS OF THE HEALTH WARNINGS LAW	BAN ON DECEITFUL TERMS*	BAN ON USE OF FIGURATIVE OR OTHER SIGNS, INCLUDING COLOURS OR NUMBERS	BAN ON PACKAGING AND LABELLING USING DESCRIPTORS DEPICTING FLAVOURS	BAN ON DISPLAY OF QUANTITATIVE INFORMATION ON EMISSION YIELDS (SUCH AS TAR, NICOTINE AND CARBON MONOXIDE)	QUIT LINE NUMBER REQUIRED TO APPEAR ON ALL PACKAGING OR LABELLING	DOES THE LAW MANDATE PLAIN PACKAGING?
Yes	Yes	No	No	No	No	No	No
No	No	Yes	No	No	No	No	No
No	Yes	No	No	No	No	No	No
Yes	Yes	Yes	Yes	No	No	No	No
No	Yes	No	No	No	No	No	No
No	Yes ⊕	Yes ⊕	Yes ⊕	No	No	No	No
No	Yes	No	No	No	No	No	No
Yes	No	No	Yes	No	No	No	No
Yes	Yes	No	No	No	Yes	No	No
Yes	Yes	Yes	No	No	No	Yes	No
No	Yes	No	No	No	No	No	No

Europe

Table 2.2.4
Additional characteristics of health warning labels on cigarette packages in Europe

Please refer to page 130 for country-specific notes.

* Terms including, but not limited to, "low tar", "light", "ultra light" or "mild", in any language.

... Data not reported/not available.

⊙ Policy adopted but not implemented by 31 December 2010.

COUNTRY	OTHER REQUIREMENTS FOR HEALTH WARNING LABELS ON PACKAGES		
	WARNING MUST BE PLACED AT THE TOP OF THE PRINCIPAL DISPLAY AREA	WARNINGS MUST NOT REMOVE OR DIMINISH THE LIABILITY OF THE TOBACCO INDUSTRY	LAW APPLIES TO PRODUCTS WHETHER MANUFACTURED DOMESTICALLY, IMPORTED, OR FOR DUTY-FREE SALE
Albania	No	No	No
Andorra[3]	...	...	...
Armenia	No	No	Yes
Austria	No	No	Yes
Azerbaijan	No	No	No
Belarus	No	No	Yes
Belgium	No	No	Yes
Bosnia and Herzegovina[4]	...	...	...
Bulgaria	No	No	Yes
Croatia	No	No	...
Cyprus	No	No	Yes
Czech Republic	No	No	Yes
Denmark	No	No	Yes
Estonia	No	No	Yes
Finland	No	No	Yes
France	No	No	Yes
Georgia	No	No	Yes
Germany	No	No	Yes
Greece	No	No	Yes
Hungary	No	No	Yes
Iceland	No	No	Yes
Ireland	No	No	Yes
Israel	No	No	Yes
Italy	Yes	No	Yes
Kazakhstan	No	No	No
Kyrgyzstan	No	No	No
Latvia	No	No	No
Lithuania	No	No	Yes
Luxembourg	No	No	Yes
Malta	No	No	Yes
Monaco[6]	...	...	...
Montenegro	No	No	Yes
Netherlands	No	No	Yes
Norway	No	No	Yes
Poland	No	No	Yes
Portugal	Yes	No	Yes
Republic of Moldova	No	No	Yes
Romania	No	No	Yes
Russian Federation	No	No	Yes
San Marino	No	No	No
Serbia	No	No	Yes
Slovakia	No	No	Yes
Slovenia	No	No	No
Spain	No	No	Yes
Sweden	No	No	No
Switzerland	No	No	Yes
Tajikistan	No	No	No
The former Yugoslav Republic of Macedonia	No	No	Yes
Turkey	No	No	Yes
Turkmenistan	No	No	No
Ukraine	No	No	Yes
United Kingdom of Great Britain and Northern Ireland	No	No	Yes
Uzbekistan	No	No	Yes

mpower

OTHER REQUIREMENTS FOR HEALTH WARNING LABELS ON PACKAGES		OTHER RESTRICTIONS REGARDING PACKAGING					
WARNINGS MUST NOT BE OBSCURED IN ANY WAY, INCLUDING BY REQUIRED MARKINGS SUCH AS TAX STAMPS	LAW REQUIRES OR ESTABLISHES FINES FOR VIOLATIONS OF THE HEALTH WARNINGS LAW	BAN ON DECEITFUL TERMS*	BAN ON USE OF FIGURATIVE OR OTHER SIGNS, INCLUDING COLOURS OR NUMBERS	BAN ON PACKAGING AND LABELLING USING DESCRIPTORS DEPICTING FLAVOURS	BAN ON DISPLAY OF QUANTITATIVE INFORMATION ON EMISSION YIELDS (SUCH AS TAR, NICOTINE AND CARBON MONOXIDE)	QUIT LINE NUMBER REQUIRED TO APPEAR ON ALL PACKAGING OR LABELLING	DOES THE LAW MANDATE PLAIN PACKAGING?
Yes	Yes	Yes	Yes	No	No	No	No
...	...	...	...	...	...	...	...
Yes	No	Yes	No	No	No	No	No
Yes	Yes	Yes	Yes	No	No	No	No
Yes	No	No	No	No	No	No	No
Yes	Yes	Yes	No	No	No	No	No
Yes	Yes	Yes	Yes	No	No	Yes	No
...	...	...	...	...	...	...	...
Yes	Yes	Yes	Yes	No	No	No	No
Yes	Yes	Yes	Yes	No	No	No	No
Yes	Yes	Yes	Yes	No	No	No	No
Yes	Yes	Yes	Yes	No	No	No	No
Yes	Yes	Yes	Yes	No	No	No[5]	No
Yes	No	Yes	Yes	No	No	No	No
Yes	Yes	Yes	Yes	No	No	No	No
Yes	Yes	Yes	Yes	No	No	Yes	No
Yes	Yes	Yes	Yes	No	No	Yes	No
Yes	Yes	Yes	Yes	No	No	No	No
Yes	Yes	Yes	No	No	No	No	No
Yes	Yes	Yes	Yes	No	No	No	No
Yes	Yes	Yes	Yes	No	No	No	No
Yes	Yes	Yes	Yes	No	No	No	No
No	Yes	Yes	Yes	No	No	No	No
Yes	Yes	Yes	Yes	No	No	No	No
No	No	Yes	No	No	No	No	No
Yes	Yes	Yes	No	No	No	Yes	No
Yes	Yes	Yes	Yes	No	No	No	No
Yes	Yes	Yes	Yes	No	No	No	No
Yes	Yes	Yes	Yes	No	No	No	No
Yes	Yes	Yes	Yes	No	No	No	No
...	...	...	...	...	...	...	...
Yes	Yes	Yes	No	No	No	No	No
Yes	No	Yes	Yes	No	No	No	No
Yes	Yes	Yes	Yes	No	No	Yes	No
Yes	Yes	Yes	Yes	No	No	No	No
Yes	Yes	Yes	Yes	No	No	No	No
No	No	Yes	Yes	No	No	No	No
Yes	Yes	Yes	Yes	No	No	No	No
No	Yes	No	No	No	No	No	No
No	No	...	...	...	...	...	...
No	Yes	Yes	No	No	No	No	No
Yes	Yes	Yes	Yes	No	No	No	No
Yes	Yes	Yes	Yes	No	No	Yes	No
Yes	Yes	Yes	Yes	No	No	No	No
Yes	Yes	Yes	Yes	No	No	No	No
No	Yes	Yes	Yes	No	No	Yes	No
No	No	...	...	...	...	...	...
Yes	No	Yes	Yes	No	No	No	No
Yes	Yes	Yes	Yes	No	No	No	No
No	No	...	...	...	...	...	...
Yes[6]	Yes	Yes	Yes	No	No	No	No
Yes	Yes	Yes	Yes	No	No	No	No
No	No	No	No	No	No	No	No

Eastern Mediterranean

Table 2.2.5
Additional characteristics of health warning labels on cigarette packages in the Eastern Mediterranean

Please refer to page 130 for country-specific notes.

* Terms including, but not limited to, "low tar", "light", "ultra light" or "mild", in any language.

< Refers to a territory.

COUNTRY	OTHER REQUIREMENTS FOR HEALTH WARNING LABELS ON PACKAGES		
	WARNING MUST BE PLACED AT THE TOP OF THE PRINCIPAL DISPLAY AREA	WARNINGS MUST NOT REMOVE OR DIMINISH THE LIABILITY OF THE TOBACCO INDUSTRY	LAW APPLIES TO PRODUCTS WHETHER MANUFACTURED DOMESTICALLY, IMPORTED, OR FOR DUTY-FREE SALE
Afghanistan	No	No	No
Bahrain	No	No	No
Djibouti	Yes	Yes	Yes
Egypt	No	No	Yes
Iran (Islamic Republic of)	Yes	No	No
Iraq	No	No	Yes
Jordan	No	No	Yes
Kuwait	No	No	Yes
Lebanon	No	No	Yes
Libyan Arab Jamahiriya	No	No	Yes
Morocco	No	No	No
Oman	No	No	No
Pakistan	Yes	No	Yes
Qatar	No	No	Yes
Saudi Arabia	No	No	No
Somalia	No	No	No
Sudan	No	No	Yes
Syrian Arab Republic	No	No	Yes
Tunisia	No	No	No
United Arab Emirates	No	No	No
West Bank and Gaza Strip<	No	No	Yes
Yemen	No	No	Yes

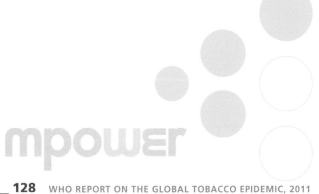

OTHER REQUIREMENTS FOR HEALTH WARNING LABELS ON PACKAGES		OTHER RESTRICTIONS REGARDING PACKAGING					
WARNINGS MUST NOT BE OBSCURED IN ANY WAY, INCLUDING BY REQUIRED MARKINGS SUCH AS TAX STAMPS	LAW REQUIRES OR ESTABLISHES FINES FOR VIOLATIONS OF THE HEALTH WARNINGS LAW	BAN ON DECEITFUL TERMS*	BAN ON USE OF FIGURATIVE OR OTHER SIGNS, INCLUDING COLOURS OR NUMBERS	BAN ON PACKAGING AND LABELLING USING DESCRIPTORS DEPICTING FLAVOURS	BAN ON DISPLAY OF QUANTITATIVE INFORMATION ON EMISSION YIELDS (SUCH AS TAR, NICOTINE AND CARBON MONOXIDE)	QUIT LINE NUMBER REQUIRED TO APPEAR ON ALL PACKAGING OR LABELLING	DOES THE LAW MANDATE PLAIN PACKAGING?
No	No	No	No	No	No	No	No
No	No	No	No	No	No	No	No
Yes	Yes	Yes	Yes	No	No	No	No
No	Yes	Yes	No	No	No	No	No
No	No	Yes	No	No	No	No	No
No	No	No	No	No	No	No	No
No	Yes	No	No	No	No	No	No
Yes	No	No	No	No	No	No	No
No	Yes	No	No	No	No	No	No
No	No	No	No	No	No	No	No
No	Yes	No	No	No	No	No	No
No	Yes	No	No	No	No	No	No
No	Yes	No	No	No	No	No	No
No	Yes	No	No	No	No	No	No
No	No	No	No	No	No	No	No
No	No	No	No	No	No	No	No
No	Yes	No	No	No	No	No	No
No	Yes	No	No	No	No	No	No
No	Yes	No	No	No	No	No	No
No	Yes	No	No	No	No	No	No
No	Yes	No	No	No	No	No	No
No	Yes	No	No	No	No	No	No

Western Pacific

Table 2.2.6
Additional characteristics of health warning labels on cigarette packages in the Western Pacific

* Terms including, but not limited to, "low tar", "light", "ultra light" or "mild", in any language.

⊙ Policy adopted but not implemented by 31 December 2010.

. . . Data not reported/not available.

NOTES TO APPENDIX II TABLE 2.2

1 Regulations will be issued shortly.

2 Bhutan prohibits the sale of all tobacco products; tobacco products imported for personal consumption shall show the country of origin and appropriate health warnings as required by the Ministry of Health.

3 All tobacco products sold in Andorra are imported from France or Spain and therefore follow the French or Spanish laws on health warnings.

4 The two subnational jurisdictions of the country, Federation of Bosnia and Herzegovina and Republika Srpska, adopted separate tobacco control legislation with several differences, so no national legislation is reported.

5 In Denmark, the quit line number appears on one of the 16 rotating health warnings.

6 All tobacco products sold in Monaco are imported from France and therefore follow the French law on health warnings.

7 It is mandatory that a website address appears on the package providing information about smoking cessation.

COUNTRY	OTHER REQUIREMENTS FOR HEALTH WARNING LABELS ON PACKAGES		
	WARNING MUST BE PLACED AT THE TOP OF THE PRINCIPAL DISPLAY AREA	WARNINGS MUST NOT REMOVE OR DIMINISH THE LIABILITY OF THE TOBACCO INDUSTRY	LAW APPLIES TO PRODUCTS WHETHER MANUFACTURED DOMESTICALLY, IMPORTED, OR FOR DUTY-FREE SALE
Australia	Yes	No	No
Brunei Darussalam	Yes	No	Yes
Cambodia	No	No	No
China	No	No	Yes
Cook Islands	Yes	No	Yes
Fiji	No	No	No
Japan	No	No	Yes
Kiribati	. . .	. . .	. . .
Lao People's Democratic Republic	Yes	No	Yes
Malaysia	Yes	No	Yes
Marshall Islands	No	Yes	Yes
Micronesia (Federated States of)	No	No	No
Mongolia	No	No	Yes
Nauru	No	No	Yes
New Zealand	Yes	No	Yes
Niue	No	No	No
Palau	No	No	No
Papua New Guinea	. . .	No	Yes
Philippines	Yes	No	Yes
Republic of Korea	No	No	Yes
Samoa	No	Yes	Yes
Singapore	Yes	No	No
Solomon Islands	No	No	Yes ⊙
Tonga	No	No	Yes
Tuvalu	No	Yes	Yes
Vanuatu	No	No	Yes
Viet Nam	No	No	No

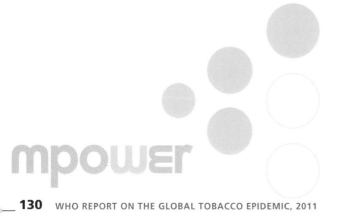

OTHER REQUIREMENTS FOR HEALTH WARNING LABELS ON PACKAGES		OTHER RESTRICTIONS REGARDING PACKAGING					
WARNINGS MUST NOT BE OBSCURED IN ANY WAY, INCLUDING BY REQUIRED MARKINGS SUCH AS TAX STAMPS	LAW REQUIRES OR ESTABLISHES FINES FOR VIOLATIONS OF THE HEALTH WARNINGS LAW	BAN ON DECEITFUL TERMS*	BAN ON USE OF FIGURATIVE OR OTHER SIGNS, INCLUDING COLOURS OR NUMBERS	BAN ON PACKAGING AND LABELLING USING DESCRIPTORS DEPICTING FLAVOURS	BAN ON DISPLAY OF QUANTITATIVE INFORMATION ON EMISSION YIELDS (SUCH AS TAR, NICOTINE AND CARBON MONOXIDE)	QUIT LINE NUMBER REQUIRED TO APPEAR ON ALL PACKAGING OR LABELLING	DOES THE LAW MANDATE PLAIN PACKAGING?
Yes	Yes	Yes	Yes	Yes	Yes	Yes	No
Yes	Yes	No	No	No	Yes	No	No
No	No	No	No	No	No	No	No
No	Yes	Yes	No	No	No	No	No
Yes	Yes	Yes	Yes	No	No	No	No
No	No	No	No	No	No	No	No
Yes	Yes	No	No	No	No	No[7]	No
...	...	...	...	...	...	...	...
No	Yes	Yes	No	No	No	No	No
Yes	Yes	Yes	Yes	No	No	Yes	No
No	Yes	No	No	No	No	No	No
No	No	No	No	No	No	No	No
No	Yes	Yes	Yes	No	No	No	No
Yes	No	No	No	No	No	No	No
Yes	Yes	No	No	No	No	Yes	No
No	No	No	No	No	No	No	No
No	No	No	No	No	No	No	No
...	Yes	...	...	...	No	...	...
Yes	Yes	Yes	Yes	No	No	No	No
No	Yes	No	No	No	No	No	No
No	Yes	Yes	Yes	No	No	No	No
Yes	Yes	Yes	Yes	No	No	Yes	No
Yes ®	Yes ®	Yes ®	Yes ®	No	No	No	No
No	Yes	No	No	No	No	No	No
Yes	Yes	Yes	No	No	No	No	No
No	Yes	Yes	No	No	No	No	No
No	Yes	No	No	No	No	No	No

Africa

Table 2.3.1
Anti-tobacco mass media campaigns in Africa

* A campaign is a communication activity lasting at least one three-week period during a year, which utilizes mass media (television, radio, print, outdoor billboards, Internet) to inform and educate the public about the harms of tobacco use and second-hand smoke exposure, to increase support for tobacco control policies or laws, to encourage tobacco users to quit, and/or to challenge tobacco industry practices.

. . . Data not reported/not available.

— Data not required/not applicable

COUNTRY	DID THE COUNTRY HAVE AT LEAST ONE NATIONAL MASS MEDIA CAMPAIGN DURING 2009 OR 2010?*
Algeria	No
Angola	No
Benin	No
Botswana	Yes
Burkina Faso	No
Burundi	No
Cameroon	No
Cape Verde	No
Central African Republic	No
Chad	No
Comoros	No
Congo	No
Côte d'Ivoire	Yes
Democratic Republic of the Congo	. . .
Equatorial Guinea	No
Eritrea	Yes
Ethiopia	No
Gabon	. . .
Gambia	No
Ghana	No
Guinea	Yes
Guinea-Bissau	No
Kenya	No
Lesotho	No
Liberia	No
Madagascar	Yes
Malawi	No
Mali	No
Mauritania	. . .
Mauritius	No
Mozambique	No
Namibia	No
Niger	Yes
Nigeria	No
Rwanda	Yes
Sao Tome and Principe	No
Senegal	No
Seychelles	Yes
Sierra Leone	No
South Africa	No
Swaziland	No
Togo	Yes
Uganda	No
United Republic of Tanzania	No
Zambia	Yes
Zimbabwe	No

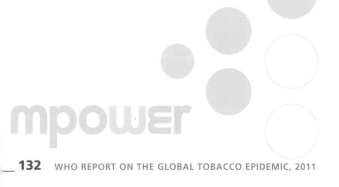

mpower

EVIDENCE-BASED PLANNING			IMPLEMENTATION		EVALUATION	
CAMPAIGN WAS PART OF A COMPREHENSIVE TOBACCO CONTROL PROGRAMME	CAMPAIGN WAS PRE-TESTED	FORMATIVE RESEARCH WAS CONDUCTED	CAMPAIGN UTILIZED MEDIA PLANNING	EARNED MEDIA/ PUBLIC RELATIONS WERE USED TO PROMOTE THE CAMPAIGN	PROCESS EVALUATION WAS EMPLOYED TO ASSESS IMPLEMENTATION	OUTCOME EVALUATION WAS EMPLOYED TO ASSESS EFFECTIVENESS
—	—	—	—	—	—	—
—	—	—	—	—	—	—
—	—	—	—	—	—	—
Yes	No	Yes	Yes	Yes	No	No
—	—	—	—	—	—	—
—	—	—	—	—	—	—
—	—	—	—	—	—	—
—	—	—	—	—	—	—
—	—	—	—	—	—	—
—	—	—	—	—	—	—
—	—	—	—	—	—	—
Yes	No	No	Yes	Yes	No	No
...	...	...	...	...	...	...
—	—	—	—	—	—	—
Yes	No	Yes	Yes	Yes	Yes	No
—	—	—	—	—	—	—
...	...	...	...	...	...	...
—	—	—	—	—	—	—
—	—	—	—	—	—	—
Yes	No	Yes	Yes	Yes	No	No
—	—	—	—	—	—	—
—	—	—	—	—	—	—
—	—	—	—	—	—	—
—	—	—	—	—	—	—
Yes	Yes	Yes	Yes	Yes	Yes	No
—	—	—	—	—	—	—
—	—	—	—	—	—	—
...	...	...	...	...	...	...
—	—	—	—	—	—	—
—	—	—	—	—	—	—
—	—	—	—	—	—	—
Yes	Yes	Yes	Yes	Yes	Yes	Yes
—	—	—	—	—	—	—
Yes	No	Yes	Yes	Yes	Yes	Yes
—	—	—	—	—	—	—
—	—	—	—	—	—	—
Yes	No	No	Yes	Yes	Yes	No
—	—	—	—	—	—	—
—	—	—	—	—	—	—
—	—	—	—	—	—	—
Yes	No	Yes	Yes	Yes	Yes	Yes
—	—	—	—	—	—	—
—	—	—	—	—	—	—
Yes	Yes	Yes	Yes	Yes	Yes	No
—	—	—	—	—	—	—

The Americas

Table 2.3.2
Anti-tobacco mass media campaigns in the Americas

Please refer to page 142 for country-specific notes.

*   A campaign is a communication activity lasting at least one three-week period during a year, which utilizes mass media (television, radio, print, outdoor billboards, Internet) to inform and educate the public about the harms of tobacco use and second-hand smoke exposure, to increase support for tobacco control policies or laws, to encourage tobacco users to quit, and/or to challenge tobacco industry practices.

... Data not reported/not available.

— Data not required/not applicable

COUNTRY	DID THE COUNTRY HAVE AT LEAST ONE NATIONAL MASS MEDIA CAMPAIGN DURING 2009 OR 2010?*
Antigua and Barbuda	...
Argentina	Yes
Bahamas	No
Barbados	Yes
Belize	No
Bolivia (Plurinational State of)	No
Brazil	Yes
Canada[1]	No
Chile	No
Colombia	Yes
Costa Rica	No
Cuba	Yes
Dominica	...
Dominican Republic	No
Ecuador[2]	No
El Salvador	Yes
Grenada	No
Guatemala	No
Guyana	No
Haiti	...
Honduras	Yes
Jamaica	No
Mexico	No
Nicaragua	No
Panama	No
Paraguay	No
Peru	No
Saint Kitts and Nevis	No
Saint Lucia	No
Saint Vincent and the Grenadines	...
Suriname	No
Trinidad and Tobago	...
United States of America	No
Uruguay	Yes
Venezuela (Bolivarian Republic of)	Yes

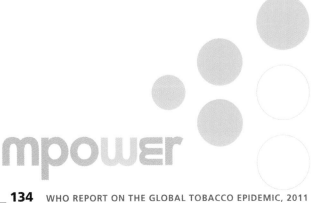

mpower

EVIDENCE-BASED PLANNING			IMPLEMENTATION		EVALUATION	
CAMPAIGN WAS PART OF A COMPREHENSIVE TOBACCO CONTROL PROGRAMME	CAMPAIGN WAS PRE-TESTED	FORMATIVE RESEARCH WAS CONDUCTED	CAMPAIGN UTILIZED MEDIA PLANNING	EARNED MEDIA/ PUBLIC RELATIONS WERE USED TO PROMOTE THE CAMPAIGN	PROCESS EVALUATION WAS EMPLOYED TO ASSESS IMPLEMENTATION	OUTCOME EVALUATION WAS EMPLOYED TO ASSESS EFFECTIVENESS
...	...	...	...	...	...	...
Yes	No	Yes	Yes	Yes	Yes	No
—	—	—	—	—	—	—
Yes	Yes	Yes	Yes	Yes	Yes	No
—	—	—	—	—	—	—
—	—	—	—	—	—	—
Yes	No	No	Yes	Yes	Yes	No
—	—	—	—	—	—	—
—	—	—	—	—	—	—
No	Yes	Yes	Yes	Yes	Yes	Yes
—	—	—	—	—	—	—
Yes	Yes	Yes	Yes	Yes	Yes	Yes
...	...	...	...	...	...	...
—	—	—	—	—	—	—
—	—	—	—	—	—	—
No	No	Yes	Yes	Yes	Yes	Yes
—	—	—	—	—	—	—
—	—	—	—	—	—	—
...	...	...	...	...	...	...
No	No	Yes	Yes	Yes	Yes	No
—	—	—	—	—	—	—
—	—	—	—	—	—	—
—	—	—	—	—	—	—
—	—	—	—	—	—	—
—	—	—	—	—	—	—
—	—	—	—	—	—	—
—	—	—	—	—	—	—
...	...	...	...	...	...	...
—	—	—	—	—	—	—
...	...	...	...	...	...	...
—	—	—	—	—	—	—
Yes	No	Yes	Yes	Yes	Yes	No
Yes	No	Yes	Yes	Yes	Yes	Yes

South-East Asia

Table 2.3.3
Anti-tobacco mass media campaigns in South-East Asia

* A campaign is a communication activity lasting at least one three-week period during a year, which utilizes mass media (television, radio, print, outdoor billboards, Internet) to inform and educate the public about the harms of tobacco use and second-hand smoke exposure, to increase support for tobacco control policies or laws, to encourage tobacco users to quit, and/or to challenge tobacco industry practices.

. . . Data not reported/not available.

— Data not required/not applicable

COUNTRY	DID THE COUNTRY HAVE AT LEAST ONE NATIONAL MASS MEDIA CAMPAIGN DURING 2009 OR 2010?*
Bangladesh	No
Bhutan	Yes
Democratic People's Republic of Korea	. . .
India	Yes
Indonesia	No
Maldives	No
Myanmar	Yes
Nepal	Yes
Sri Lanka	Yes
Thailand	Yes
Timor-Leste	. . .

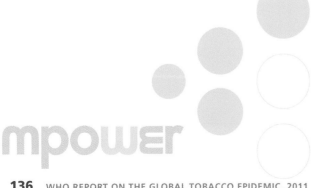

mpower

EVIDENCE-BASED PLANNING			IMPLEMENTATION		EVALUATION	
CAMPAIGN WAS PART OF A COMPREHENSIVE TOBACCO CONTROL PROGRAMME	CAMPAIGN WAS PRE-TESTED	FORMATIVE RESEARCH WAS CONDUCTED	CAMPAIGN UTILIZED MEDIA PLANNING	EARNED MEDIA/ PUBLIC RELATIONS WERE USED TO PROMOTE THE CAMPAIGN	PROCESS EVALUATION WAS EMPLOYED TO ASSESS IMPLEMENTATION	OUTCOME EVALUATION WAS EMPLOYED TO ASSESS EFFECTIVENESS
—	—	—	—	—	—	—
Yes	Yes	Yes	Yes	Yes	Yes	Yes
...	...	...	...	...	...	...
Yes	Yes	Yes	Yes	Yes	Yes	Yes
—	—	—	—	—	—	—
—	—	—	—	—	—	—
Yes	No	...	No	No	No	No
Yes	Yes	Yes	Yes	No	Yes	No
Yes	No	Yes	Yes	No	Yes	No
Yes	No	No	Yes	Yes	Yes	Yes
...	...	...	...	...	...	...

Europe

Table 2.3.4
Anti-tobacco mass media campaigns in Europe

Please refer to page 142 for country-specific notes.

* A campaign is a communication activity lasting at least one three-week period during a year, which utilizes mass media (television, radio, print, outdoor billboards, Internet) to inform and educate the public about the harms of tobacco use and second-hand smoke exposure, to increase support for tobacco control policies or laws, to encourage tobacco users to quit, and/or to challenge tobacco industry practices.

... Data not reported/not available.

— Data not required/not applicable

COUNTRY	DID THE COUNTRY HAVE AT LEAST ONE NATIONAL MASS MEDIA CAMPAIGN DURING 2009 OR 2010?*
Albania	Yes
Andorra	...
Armenia	No
Austria	No
Azerbaijan	No
Belarus	No
Belgium	No
Bosnia and Herzegovina	No
Bulgaria	No
Croatia	No
Cyprus	...
Czech Republic	Yes
Denmark	Yes
Estonia	...
Finland	Yes
France	Yes
Georgia	Yes
Germany	Yes
Greece	Yes
Hungary	Yes
Iceland	No
Ireland	Yes
Israel	Yes
Italy	Yes
Kazakhstan	Yes
Kyrgyzstan	No
Latvia	No
Lithuania	No
Luxembourg	...
Malta	Yes
Monaco	...
Montenegro	No
Netherlands	Yes
Norway	No
Poland	Yes
Portugal	No
Republic of Moldova	Yes
Romania	Yes
Russian Federation	Yes
San Marino	...
Serbia	Yes
Slovakia	No
Slovenia	No
Spain	No
Sweden	Yes
Switzerland	Yes
Tajikistan	No
The former Yugoslav Republic of Macedonia	...
Turkey	Yes
Turkmenistan	...
Ukraine	No
United Kingdom of Great Britain and Northern Ireland[3]	Yes
Uzbekistan	No

mpower

	EVIDENCE-BASED PLANNING			IMPLEMENTATION		EVALUATION	
CAMPAIGN WAS PART OF A COMPREHENSIVE TOBACCO CONTROL PROGRAMME	CAMPAIGN WAS PRE-TESTED	FORMATIVE RESEARCH WAS CONDUCTED	CAMPAIGN UTILIZED MEDIA PLANNING	EARNED MEDIA/ PUBLIC RELATIONS WERE USED TO PROMOTE THE CAMPAIGN	PROCESS EVALUATION WAS EMPLOYED TO ASSESS IMPLEMENTATION	OUTCOME EVALUATION WAS EMPLOYED TO ASSESS EFFECTIVENESS
Yes	Yes	Yes	Yes	Yes	No	Yes
…	…	…	…	…	…	…
—	—	—	—	—	—	—
—	—	—	—	—	—	—
—	—	—	—	—	—	—
—	—	—	—	—	—	—
—	—	—	—	—	—	—
—	—	—	—	—	—	—
—	—	—	—	—	—	—
…	…	…	…	…	…	…
No	Yes	…	Yes	Yes	Yes	Yes
Yes	Yes	Yes	Yes	Yes	Yes	Yes
…	…	…	…	…	…	…
Yes	No	Yes	Yes	Yes	Yes	Yes
No	No	No	Yes	Yes	No	Yes
Yes	No	Yes	Yes	Yes	No	Yes
No	Yes	Yes	Yes	Yes	Yes	Yes
Yes	Yes	Yes	Yes	Yes	Yes	Yes
No	No	…	No	Yes	No	No
—	—	—	—	—	—	—
Yes	Yes	Yes	Yes	Yes	Yes	Yes
No	No	Yes	Yes	Yes	Yes	Yes
Yes	No	Yes	Yes	No	Yes	Yes
Yes	Yes	Yes	Yes	Yes	Yes	No
—	—	—	—	—	—	—
—	—	—	—	—	—	—
—	—	—	—	—	—	—
…	…	…	…	…	…	…
Yes	No	Yes	Yes	Yes	Yes	No
…	…	…	…	…	…	…
—	—	—	—	—	—	—
Yes	Yes	Yes	Yes	Yes	Yes	Yes
—	—	—	—	—	—	—
Yes	No	Yes	Yes	Yes	Yes	Yes
—	—	—	—	—	—	—
No	No	No	Yes	Yes	Yes	No
Yes	No	…	Yes	Yes	No	Yes
Yes	Yes	Yes	Yes	Yes	Yes	Yes
…	…	…	…	…	…	…
Yes	Yes	Yes	Yes	Yes	Yes	Yes
—	—	—	—	—	—	—
—	—	—	—	—	—	—
Yes	Yes	Yes	Yes	Yes	Yes	Yes
Yes	No	Yes	Yes	Yes	Yes	Yes
—	—	—	—	—	—	—
…	…	…	…	…	…	…
Yes	Yes	Yes	Yes	Yes	Yes	Yes
…	…	…	…	…	…	…
—	—	—	—	—	—	—
Yes	Yes	Yes	Yes	Yes	Yes	Yes
—	—	—	—	—	—	—

Eastern Mediterranean

Table 2.3.5
Anti-tobacco mass media campaigns in the Eastern Mediterranean

* A campaign is a communication activity lasting at least one three-week period during a year, which utilizes mass media (television, radio, print, outdoor billboards, Internet) to inform and educate the public about the harms of tobacco use and second-hand smoke exposure, to increase support for tobacco control policies or laws, to encourage tobacco users to quit, and/or to challenge tobacco industry practices.

... Data not reported/not available.

— Data not required/not applicable

< Refers to a territory.

COUNTRY	DID THE COUNTRY HAVE AT LEAST ONE NATIONAL MASS MEDIA CAMPAIGN DURING 2009 OR 2010?*
Afghanistan	...
Bahrain	Yes
Djibouti	No
Egypt	Yes
Iran (Islamic Republic of)	...
Iraq	No
Jordan	Yes
Kuwait	Yes
Lebanon	Yes
Libyan Arab Jamahiriya	No
Morocco	Yes
Oman	No
Pakistan	No
Qatar	No
Saudi Arabia	Yes
Somalia	...
Sudan	Yes
Syrian Arab Republic	...
Tunisia	Yes
United Arab Emirates	Yes
West Bank and Gaza Strip<	No
Yemen	Yes

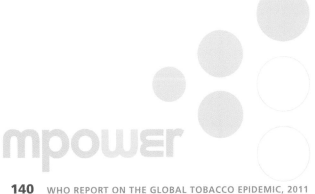

EVIDENCE-BASED PLANNING			IMPLEMENTATION		EVALUATION	
CAMPAIGN WAS PART OF A COMPREHENSIVE TOBACCO CONTROL PROGRAMME	CAMPAIGN WAS PRE-TESTED	FORMATIVE RESEARCH WAS CONDUCTED	CAMPAIGN UTILIZED MEDIA PLANNING	EARNED MEDIA/ PUBLIC RELATIONS WERE USED TO PROMOTE THE CAMPAIGN	PROCESS EVALUATION WAS EMPLOYED TO ASSESS IMPLEMENTATION	OUTCOME EVALUATION WAS EMPLOYED TO ASSESS EFFECTIVENESS
...	...	...	...	...	...	...
Yes	No	Yes	Yes	Yes	Yes	No
—	—	—	—	—	—	—
Yes	Yes	Yes	Yes	Yes	Yes	Yes
...	...	...	...	...	...	...
—	—	—	—	—	—	—
Yes	No	Yes	Yes	Yes	Yes	No
Yes	Yes	No	Yes	Yes	Yes	No
Yes	Yes	Yes	Yes	Yes	Yes	Yes
—	—	—	—	—	—	—
Yes	Yes	Yes	Yes	Yes	Yes	Yes
—	—	—	—	—	—	—
—	—	—	—	—	—	—
—	—	—	—	—	—	—
Yes	No	No	Yes	Yes	No	...
...	...	...	...	...	...	...
Yes	No	Yes	Yes	Yes	No	No
...	...	...	...	...	...	...
Yes	No	Yes	Yes	Yes	No	No
Yes	No	Yes	No	Yes	Yes	No
—	—	—	—	—	—	—
No	No	Yes	Yes	Yes	No	No

Western Pacific

Table 2.3.6
Anti-tobacco mass media campaigns in the Western Pacific

* A campaign is a communication activity lasting at least one three-week period during a year, which utilizes mass media (television, radio, print, outdoor billboards, Internet) to inform and educate the public about the harms of tobacco use and second-hand smoke exposure, to increase support for tobacco control policies or laws, to encourage tobacco users to quit, and/or to challenge tobacco industry practices.

… Data not reported/not available.

— Data not required/not applicable

NOTES TO APPENDIX II TABLE 2.3

1. The Government of Canada did not implement a nationwide mass media campaign during the reporting period. However, mass media campaigns have been implemented in eight of Canada's subnational jurisdictions.

2. There was no nationwide mass media campaign in Ecuador during the reporting period. However, mass media campaigns have been implemented in many of Ecuador's large cities.

3. Anti-tobacco mass media campaigns with similar characteristics were implemented in all four countries of the United Kingdom of Great Britain and Northern Ireland.

COUNTRY	DID THE COUNTRY HAVE AT LEAST ONE NATIONAL MASS MEDIA CAMPAIGN DURING 2009 OR 2010?*
Australia	Yes
Brunei Darussalam	Yes
Cambodia	Yes
China	No
Cook Islands	No
Fiji	No
Japan	No
Kiribati	No
Lao People's Democratic Republic	No
Malaysia	Yes
Marshall Islands	No
Micronesia (Federated States of)	No
Mongolia	Yes
Nauru	…
New Zealand	Yes
Niue	Yes
Palau	No
Papua New Guinea	No
Philippines	Yes
Republic of Korea	…
Samoa	Yes
Singapore	Yes
Solomon Islands	…
Tonga	No
Tuvalu	No
Vanuatu	…
Viet Nam	Yes

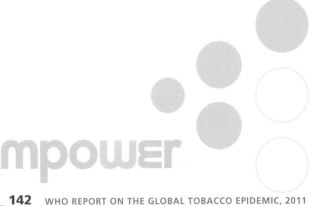

EVIDENCE-BASED PLANNING			IMPLEMENTATION		EVALUATION	
CAMPAIGN WAS PART OF A COMPREHENSIVE TOBACCO CONTROL PROGRAMME	CAMPAIGN WAS PRE-TESTED	FORMATIVE RESEARCH WAS CONDUCTED	CAMPAIGN UTILIZED MEDIA PLANNING	EARNED MEDIA/ PUBLIC RELATIONS WERE USED TO PROMOTE THE CAMPAIGN	PROCESS EVALUATION WAS EMPLOYED TO ASSESS IMPLEMENTATION	OUTCOME EVALUATION WAS EMPLOYED TO ASSESS EFFECTIVENESS
Yes	Yes	Yes	Yes	No	Yes	Yes
Yes	Yes	No	Yes	Yes	Yes	No
Yes	Yes	Yes	Yes	Yes	Yes	Yes
—	—	—	—	—	—	—
—	—	—	—	—	—	—
—	—	—	—	—	—	—
—	—	—	—	—	—	—
—	—	—	—	—	—	—
—	—	—	—	—	—	—
Yes	Yes	Yes	Yes	Yes	Yes	Yes
—	—	—	—	—	—	—
—	—	—	—	—	—	—
Yes	Yes	Yes	Yes	Yes	Yes	Yes
...	...	...	...	...	...	...
Yes	No	No	Yes	Yes	No	Yes
Yes	...	Yes	Yes	Yes	Yes	No
—	—	—	—	—	—	—
—	—	—	—	—	—	—
Yes	Yes	Yes	Yes	Yes	Yes	Yes
...	...	...	...	...	...	...
Yes	Yes	Yes	Yes	Yes	Yes	Yes
Yes	Yes	Yes	Yes	Yes	Yes	Yes
...	...	...	...	...	...	...
—	—	—	—	—	—	—
—	—	—	—	—	—	—
...	...	...	...	...	...	...
Yes	Yes	Yes	Yes	Yes	Yes	Yes

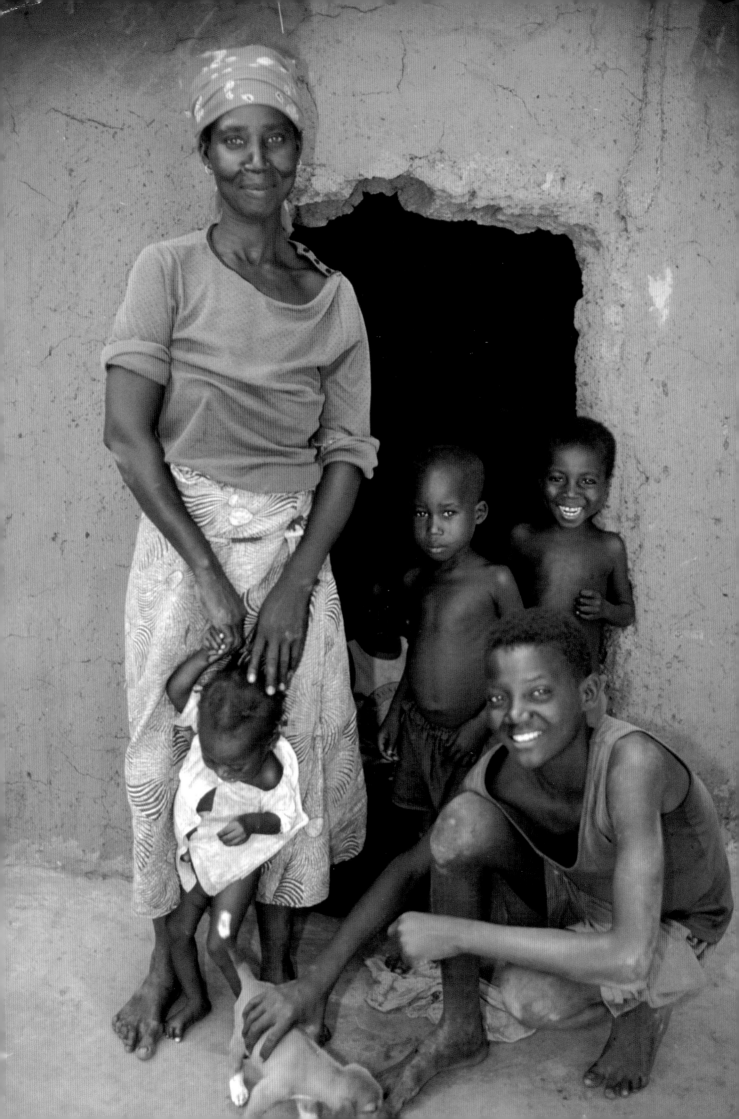

APPENDIX III: **STATUS OF THE WHO FRAMEWORK CONVENTION ON TOBACCO CONTROL**

Appendix III shows the status of the WHO Framework Convention on Tobacco Control (WHO FCTC). Ratification is the international act by which countries that have already signed a convention formally state their consent to be bound by it. Accession is the international act by which countries that have not signed a treaty/convention formally state their consent to be bound by it. Acceptance and approval are the legal equivalent of ratification. Signature of a convention indicates that a country is not legally bound by the treaty but is committed not to undermine its provisions.

The WHO FCTC entered into force on 27 February 2005, on the 90th day after the deposit of the 40th instrument of ratification in the United Nations headquarters, the depository of the treaty, in New York. The treaty remains open for ratification, acceptance, approval, formal confirmation and accession indefinitely for States and eligible regional economic integration organizations wishing to become Parties to it.

Table 3.1.0
Status of the WHO Framework Convention on Tobacco Control, as at 26 May 2011

* Ratification is the international act by which countries that have already signed a treaty or convention formally state their consent to be bound by it.

a Accession is the international act by which countries that have not signed a treaty/convention formally state their consent to be bound by it.

A Acceptance is the international act, similar to ratification, by which countries that have already signed a treaty/convention formally state their consent to be bound by it.

AA Approval is the international act, similar to ratification, by which countries that have already signed a treaty/convention formally state their consent to be bound by it.

c Formal confirmation is the international act corresponding to ratification by a State, whereby an international organization (in the case of the WHO FCTC, competent regional economic integration organizations) formally state their consent to be bound by a treaty/convention.

d Succession is the international act, however phrased or named, by which successor States formally state their consent to be bound by treaties/conventions originally entered into by their predecessor State.

COUNTRY	DATE OF SIGNATURE	DATE OF RATIFICATION* (OR LEGAL EQUIVALENT)
Afghanistan	29 June 2004	13 August 2010
Albania	29 June 2004	26 April 2006
Algeria	20 June 2003	30 June 2006
Andorra		
Angola	29 June 2004	20 September 2007
Antigua and Barbuda	28 June 2004	05 June 2006
Argentina	25 September 2003	
Armenia		29 November 2004 a
Australia	05 December 2003	27 October 2004
Austria	28 August 2003	15 September 2005
Azerbaijan		01 November 2005 a
Bahamas	29 June 2004	03 November 2009
Bahrain		20 March 2007 a
Bangladesh	16 June 2003	14 June 2004
Barbados	28 June 2004	03 November 2005
Belarus	17 June 2004	08 September 2005
Belgium	22 January 2004	01 November 2005
Belize	26 September 2003	15 December 2005
Benin	18 June 2004	03 November 2005
Bhutan	09 December 2003	23 August 2004
Bolivia (Plurinational State of)	27 February 2004	15 September 2005
Bosnia and Herzegovina		10 July 2009
Botswana	16 June 2003	31 January 2005
Brazil	16 June 2003	03 November 2005
Brunei Darussalam	03 June 2004	03 June 2004
Bulgaria	22 December 2003	07 November 2005
Burkina Faso	22 December 2003	31 July 2006
Burundi	16 June 2003	22 November 2005
Cambodia	25 May 2004	15 November 2005
Cameroon	13 May 2004	03 February 2006
Canada	15 July 2003	26 November 2004
Cape Verde	17 February 2004	04 October 2005
Central African Republic	29 December 2003	07 November 2005
Chad	22 June 2004	30 January 2006
Chile	25 September 2003	13 June 2005
China	10 November 2003	11 October 2005
Colombia		10 April 2008 a
Comoros	27 February 2004	24 January 2006
Congo	23 March 2004	06 February 2007
Cook Islands	14 May 2004	14 May 2004
Costa Rica	03 July 2003	21 August 2008
Côte d'Ivoire	24 July 2003	13 August 2010
Croatia	02 June 2004	14 July 2008
Cuba	29 June 2004	
Cyprus	24 May 2004	26 October 2005
Czech Republic	16 June 2003	
Democratic People's Republic of Korea	17 June 2003	27 April 2005
Democratic Republic of the Congo	28 June 2004	28 October 2005
Denmark	16 June 2003	16 December 2004
Djibouti	13 May 2004	31 July 2005
Dominica	29 June 2004	24 July 2006

COUNTRY	DATE OF SIGNATURE	DATE OF RATIFICATION* (OR LEGAL EQUIVALENT)
Dominican Republic		
Ecuador	22 March 2004	25 July 2006
Egypt	17 June 2003	25 February 2005
El Salvador	18 March 2004	
Equatorial Guinea		17 September 2005 [a]
Eritrea		
Estonia	08 June 2004	27 July 2005
Ethiopia	25 February 2004	
European Community	16 June 2003	30 June 2005 [c]
Fiji	03 October 2003	03 October 2003
Finland	16 June 2003	24 January 2005
France	16 June 2003	19 October 2004 [AA]
Gabon	22 August 2003	20 February 2009
Gambia	16 June 2003	18 September 2007
Georgia	20 February 2004	14 February 2006
Germany	24 October 2003	16 December 2004
Ghana	20 June 2003	29 November 2004
Greece	16 June 2003	27 January 2006
Grenada	29 June 2004	14 August 2007
Guatemala	25 September 2003	16 November 2005
Guinea	01 April 2004	07 November 2007
Guinea-Bissau		07 November 2008 [a]
Guyana		15 September 2005 [a]
Haiti	23 July 2003	
Honduras	18 June 2004	16 February 2005
Hungary	16 June 2003	07 April 2004
Iceland	16 June 2003	14 June 2004
India	10 September 2003	05 February 2004
Indonesia		
Iran (Islamic Republic of)	16 June 2003	06 November 2005
Iraq	29 June 2004	17 March 2008
Ireland	16 September 2003	07 November 2005
Israel	20 June 2003	24 August 2005
Italy	16 June 2003	02 July 2008
Jamaica	24 September 2003	07 July 2005
Japan	09 March 2004	08 June 2004 [A]
Jordan	28 May 2004	19 August 2004
Kazakhstan	21 June 2004	22 January 2007
Kenya	25 June 2004	25 June 2004
Kiribati	27 April 2004	15 September 2005
Kuwait	16 June 2003	12 May 2006
Kyrgyzstan	18 February 2004	25 May 2006
Lao People's Democratic Republic	29 June 2004	06 September 2006
Latvia	10 May 2004	10 February 2005
Lebanon	04 March 2004	07 December 2005
Lesotho	23 June 2004	14 January 2005
Liberia	25 June 2004	15 September 2009
Libyan Arab Jamahiriya	18 June 2004	07 June 2005
Lithuania	22 September 2003	16 December 2004
Luxembourg	16 June 2003	30 June 2005
Madagascar	24 September 2003	22 September 2004

Table 3.1.0
Status of the WHO Framework Convention on Tobacco Control, as at 26 May 2011

* Ratification is the international act by which countries that have already signed a treaty or convention formally state their consent to be bound by it.

a Accession is the international act by which countries that have not signed a treaty/convention formally state their consent to be bound by it.

A Acceptance is the international act, similar to ratification, by which countries that have already signed a treaty/convention formally state their consent to be bound by it.

AA Approval is the international act, similar to ratification, by which countries that have already signed a treaty/convention formally state their consent to be bound by it.

c Formal confirmation is the international act corresponding to ratification by a State, whereby an international organization (in the case of the WHO FCTC, competent regional economic integration organizations) formally state their consent to be bound by a treaty/convention.

d Succession is the international act, however phrased or named, by which successor States formally state their consent to be bound by treaties/conventions originally entered into by their predecessor State.

COUNTRY	DATE OF SIGNATURE	DATE OF RATIFICATION* (OR LEGAL EQUIVALENT)
Malawi		
Malaysia	23 September 2003	16 September 2005
Maldives	17 May 2004	20 May 2004
Mali	23 September 2003	19 October 2005
Malta	16 June 2003	24 September 2003
Marshall Islands	16 June 2003	08 December 2004
Mauritania	24 June 2004	28 October 2005
Mauritius	17 June 2003	17 May 2004
Mexico	12 August 2003	28 May 2004
Micronesia (Federated States of)	28 June 2004	18 March 2005
Monaco		
Mongolia	16 June 2003	27 January 2004
Montenegro		23 October 2006 d
Morocco	16 April 2004	
Mozambique	18 June 2003	
Myanmar	23 October 2003	21 April 2004
Namibia	29 January 2004	07 November 2005
Nauru		29 June 2004 a
Nepal	03 December 2003	07 November 2006
Netherlands	16 June 2003	27 January 2005 A
New Zealand	16 June 2003	27 January 2004
Nicaragua	07 June 2004	09 April 2008
Niger	28 June 2004	25 August 2005
Nigeria	28 June 2004	20 October 2005
Niue	18 June 2004	03 June 2005
Norway	16 June 2003	16 June 2003 AA
Oman		09 March 2005 a
Pakistan	18 May 2004	03 November 2004
Palau	16 June 2003	12 February 2004
Panama	26 September 2003	16 August 2004
Papua New Guinea	22 June 2004	25 May 2006
Paraguay	16 June 2003	26 September 2006
Peru	21 April 2004	30 November 2004
Philippines	23 September 2003	06 June 2005
Poland	14 June 2004	15 September 2006
Portugal	09 January 2004	08 November 2005 AA
Qatar	17 June 2003	23 July 2004
Republic of Korea	21 July 2003	16 May 2005
Republic of Moldova	29 June 2004	03 February 2009 a
Romania	25 June 2004	27 January 2006
Russian Federation		03 June 2008 a
Rwanda	02 June 2004	19 October 2005
Saint Kitts and Nevis	29 June 2004	
Saint Lucia	29 June 2004	07 November 2005
Saint Vincent and the Grenadines	14 June 2004	29 October 2010
Samoa	25 September 2003	03 November 2005
San Marino	26 September 2003	07 July 2004
Sao Tome and Principe	18 June 2004	12 April 2006
Saudi Arabia	24 June 2004	09 May 2005
Senegal	19 June 2003	27 January 2005
Serbia	28 June 2004	08 February 2006

COUNTRY	DATE OF SIGNATURE	DATE OF RATIFICATION* (OR LEGAL EQUIVALENT)
Seychelles	11 September 2003	12 November 2003
Sierra Leone		22 May 2009
Singapore	29 December 2003	14 May 2004
Slovakia	19 December 2003	04 May 2004
Slovenia	25 September 2003	15 March 2005
Solomon Islands	18 June 2004	10 August 2004
Somalia		
South Africa	16 June 2003	19 April 2005
Spain	16 June 2003	11 January 2005
Sri Lanka	23 September 2003	11 November 2003
Sudan	10 June 2004	31 October 2005
Suriname	24 June 2004	16 December 2008
Swaziland	29 June 2004	13 January 2006
Sweden	16 June 2003	07 July 2005
Switzerland	25 June 2004	
Syrian Arab Republic	11 July 2003	22 November 2004
Tajikistan		
Thailand	20 June 2003	08 November 2004
The former Yugoslav Republic of Macedonia		30 June 2006 ª
Timor-Leste	25 May 2004	22 December 2004
Togo	12 May 2004	15 November 2005
Tonga	25 September 2003	08 April 2005
Trinidad and Tobago	27 August 2003	19 August 2004
Tunisia	22 August 2003	07 June 2010
Turkey	28 April 2004	31 December 2004
Turkmenistan		13 May 2011
Tuvalu	10 June 2004	26 September 2005
Uganda	05 March 2004	20 June 2007
Ukraine	25 June 2004	06 June 2006
United Arab Emirates	24 June 2004	07 November 2005
United Kingdom of Great Britain and Northern Ireland	16 June 2003	16 December 2004
United Republic of Tanzania	27 January 2004	30 April 2007
United States of America	10 May 2004	
Uruguay	19 June 2003	09 September 2004
Uzbekistan		
Vanuatu	22 April 2004	16 September 2005
Venezuela (Bolivarian Republic of)	22 September 2003	27 June 2006
Viet Nam	03 September 2003	17 December 2004
Yemen	20 June 2003	22 February 2007
Zambia		23 May 2008 ª
Zimbabwe		

Source: WHO FCTC web site (http://www.who.int/fctc/signatories_parties/en/index.html, accessed 31 May 2011).

Though not a Member State of WHO, as a Member State of the United Nations, Liechtenstein is also eligible to become Party to the WHO FCTC, though it has taken no action to do so.

On submitting instruments to become Party to the WHO FCTC, some Parties have included notes and/or declarations. All notes can be viewed at http://www.who.int/fctc/signatories_parties/en/index.html. All declarations can be viewed at http://www.who.int/fctc/declarations/en/index.html.

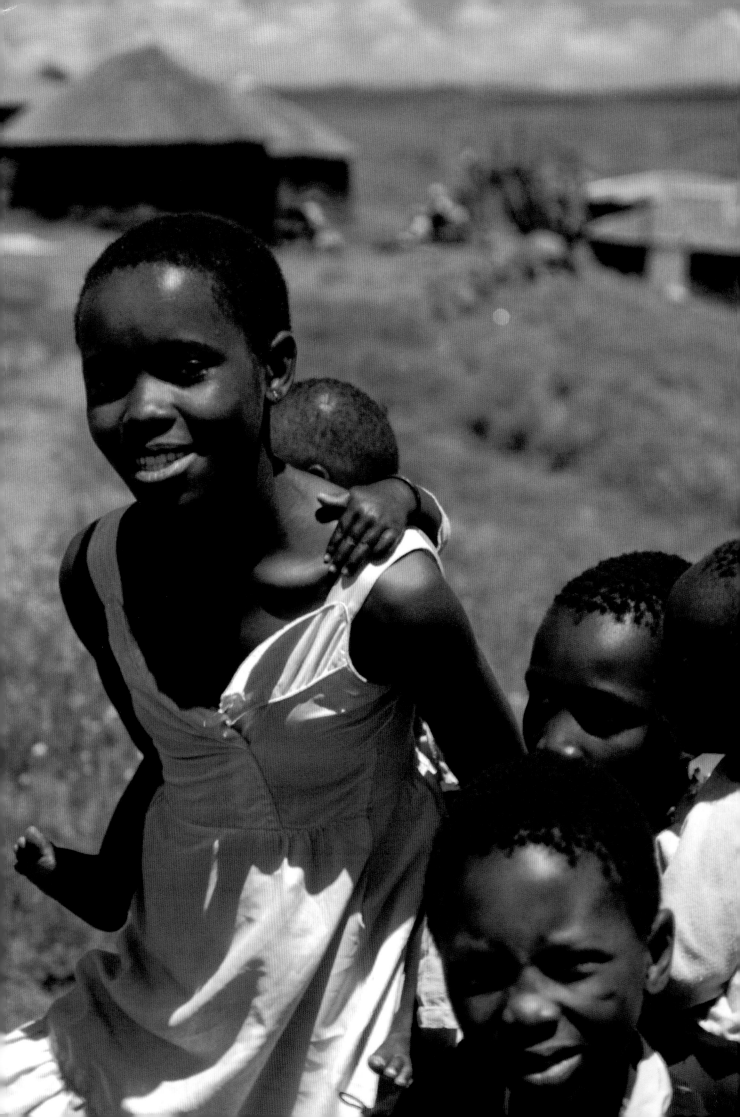

Acknowledgements

The following WHO staff assisted in compiling, analysing and editing information:

WHO African Region:
Premduth Burhoo, Tecla Butau, Deowan Mohee, Ezra Ogwell Ouma, Nivo Ramanandraibe.

WHO Region of the Americas:
Astrid Arca, Adriana Blanco, Roberta Caixeta, Rosa Sandoval, Mayte Vasquez.

WHO South-East Asia Region:
Karabi Majumdar, Dhirendra N. Sinha.

WHO European Region:
Eleni Antoniadou, Celine Brassart, Tiffany Fabro, Yulia Kadirova, Rula Khoury, Kristina Mauer-Stender, Agis Tsouros.

WHO Eastern Mediterranean Region:
Randa Abo El-Naga, Fatimah El-Awa.

WHO Western Pacific Region:
Marina Baquilod, Sarah England (China), Susan Mercado, James Rarick.

WHO-Headquarters Geneva:
Ala Alwan, Virginia Arnold, Lubna Bhatti, Douglas Bettcher, Katherine DeLand, Dongbo Fu, Raman Minhas, Timothy O'Leary, Jana Nester, Alexandre Pascutto, Armando Peruga, Vinayak Prasad, Luminita Sanda, Barbara Zolty.

Administrative support was provided by: Zahra Ali Piazza, Miriamjoy Aryee-Quansah, Gareth Burns, Catalin Iacobescu, Luis Madge, Carolyn Patten, Elizabeth Tecson, Rosane Serrao and Jennifer Volonnino.

Kerstin Schotte coordinated the production of this report. Data management, quality assurance and creation of tables, graphs and appendices were performed by Alison Commar with support from Sameer Pujari. The prevalence estimates were calculated by Gauri Khanna and Edouard Tursan d'Espaignet with help from Melanie Cowan, Hongbo Liang and Shaun Takao.

Armando Peruga was responsible for the legal review process performed by: Heather Budgell, Kayla Burns, Gemma Lien, Raman Minhas, Marine Perraudin, Jennifer Uezu, Jeremy Roth, Luminita Sanda, Julia Spitznagel, Gemma Vestal and Barbara Zolty.

The financial and economic review and analyses, including tobacco taxation and prices, were provided by Roberto Iglesias, Anne-Marle Perucic and Ayda Yurekli. Tax and price data were collected with support from officials from ministries of finance and by Matthew Allen, Murat Elibol, Christine Godwin, Luk Joossens, Konstantin Krasovsky, Aleksandra Makaj, Richard Peck, Aida Ramic-Catak, Alejandro Ramos, Deo Sekimpi and Gulnoza Usmanova.

We thank Jennifer Ellis and Kelly Henning of the Bloomberg Initiative to Reduce Tobacco Use for their collaboration.

Rob Cunningham, David Hammond and Rajeev Cherukupalli, among others, provided us with their invaluable feedback and comments, thank you very much.

Special thanks also to the Convention Secretariat to the WHO FCTC, to Colin Mathers and Gretchen Stevens, and to the team of the Office on Smoking and Health of the US Centers for Disease Control and Prevention (CDC).

We would like to thank the World Lung Foundation for their collaboration in collecting the data on anti-tobacco mass media campaigns and specifically: Jorge Alday, Mio Castillo, Claudia Cedillo, Yvette Chang, Winnie Chen, Mohamed El-Ghamrawy, Stephen Hamill, Alexey Kotov, Mego Lien, Irina Morozova, Sandra Mullin, Nandita Murukutla, Rebecca Perl, Stephan Rabimov and Kim Sebek. Tom Carroll provided valuable guidance on the development of the categorization of anti-tobacco mass media campaigns.

Drew Blakeman acted as principal drafter of this report. Special thanks are due to our copyeditor and proofreader Barbara Campanini and our designer Claude Cardot and his team for their efficiency in helping to get this report published in time.

Production of this WHO document has been supported by a grant from the World Lung Foundation with financial support from Bloomberg Philanthropies. The contents of this document are the sole responsibility of WHO and should not be regarded as reflecting the positions of the World Lung Foundation.

The *WHO Report on the Global Tobacco Epidemic, 2011* was made possible by funding from Bloomberg Philanthropies